YOUR PET ISN'T SICK

Keep MT 10/5

*10 +6
1C
42
④*

YOUR PET ISN'T SICK

He Just Wants You to Think So

HERBERT TANZER, D.V.M.

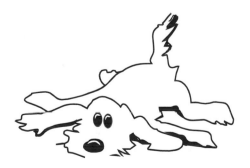

WHARTON PUBLISHING

Wharton Publishing
3790 Via de la Valle, #204
Del Mar, California 92014
(619) 756-4922

Wharton Publishing books are available for special promotions and premi-
ums. For details contact the Marketing Department at the address above.

Publisher's Cataloging-in-Publication
(Provided by Quality Books, Inc.)
  Tanzer, Herbert.
  Your pet isn't sick : (he just wants you to think so) / Herbert Tanzer. —
Rev. ed.
    p. cm.
  Preassigned LCCN: 98-87095
  ISBN: 1-56912-100-1
  1. Tanzer, Herbert. 2. Pets—Behavior. 3. Pets—Diseases. 4. Veteri-
narians—New York (State)—New York—Biography.   I. Title.
  SF412.5.T36 1998   636.089'608
                            QBI98-1080

Manufactured in the United States of America

Design: Joel Friedlander, Marin Bookworks
Editing: PeopleSpeak, Laguna Hills, CA
Cover design: Robert Aulicino / Pro-Art Graphic Design, Prescott, AZ
Illustrations (on pages 9, 15, 26, 40, 59, 86, 103, 126, 135, 162, 168,
    171): Dan Rosandich, Chassell, MI

Contents

Preface

IF THE TRUTH BE TOLD, your pet plays more games with you than you think he does. I don't mean "Catch the Ball" or "Fetch the Stick." The games I'm talking about are "Poor Baby," "Sick Dog," and "Take the Pill." These games include the full span of pet life— training, sex, disease, and relationships with owners or other pets— from the animal's earliest moments to his death.

In this book I shall let you in on some fascinating secrets that I have discovered over many years as a veterinarian. For instance, I will show you that you do not just acquire or select a pet but create it, that you are often the toy a pet plays with and manipulates, and that you can be responsible for a pet's diseases.

The case histories of pet behavior in this book are all true. The few basic concepts that are the heart of my theory—and I will repeat them many times—may be harder to believe, but the techniques do work. The cases will illustrate the "Pet Game" and your position in it. Once you understand the game, you can choose whether you wish to participate in the fun.

You may find this book revealing, amusing, challenging, or outrageous. But I very much doubt that after reading it you will ever look at any pet or relationship between a pet and its owner in the same way.

You may even find yourself, as I did, taking these ideas a step further and applying them to human animals as well. In fact, I no longer practice these techniques in a vet's office at all. Instead, I am the senior consultant of an internationally known consulting company that coaches leaders in the art of leaving their personal paw prints on the world. I spend my time dealing with two-legged animals who dress in pin-striped suits and run Fortune 500 companies and other large organizations and institutions.

How did this career change come about? I loved veterinary practice. It was rewarding in every aspect, and I could have continued to practice forever. But there were lessons I had been taught by my patients in the course of my twenty-five years of practice that I longed to share with the world. The result was my consulting work and this book. One story in particular describes a lesson I'll never forget.

An adorable five-week-old kitten was brought in to my office for her first physical examination. Fluffy encountered a cold and slippery stainless steel table to stand on, strange sounds, unusual odors, and large creatures, some with masks on, milling about. How terrifying this must have been for little Fluffy. I was behind schedule as usual, and I made the mistake of reaching too abruptly for the little patient. The absolutely terrified kitten arched her back, bristled her hair, hissed, and struck out with her needle-sharp claws at my extended hand. I can still recall the excruciating pain of one of those claws being hooked in the fleshy area between my thumb and index finger.

I had a strong desire to knock the little kitten across the room with my free hand, but I didn't. Instead, I took a deep breath, carefully unhooked the claw from my hand, picked up the little kitten by her tail, calmed her down, and then proceeded with what had to be done. What saved both of us was the realization that Fluffy wasn't mean, she was just terrified. It would be absurd for a grown man to strike a frightened kitten.

Years later I found myself dealing with a senior executive who was also being nasty. Again, I wanted to slap him, but I didn't. I stopped for a moment and imagined him covered with fur, his back arched and hair bristled while he struck out at people around him. Instead of reacting to his bad temper, I realized that underneath it was a man as frightened as the kitten had been. Once I recognized his fear, it was easy for me to calm him down and then proceed with what had to be done. At that moment I realized that the techniques I had used on animals worked wonders on people, too. My second career began and eventually led to this book.

You can read this book in two ways, on two different levels. First, it is a useful book that will help you discover some of the secrets of the Pet Game and apply them in your life with your pet. But on another level, this book is about people, and it uses pets as a metaphor to understand human behavior. This book will make you realize why your cat scratches the couch while you're at work and how you helped teach him that game. But if you also begin to see pet games like the ones in this book being played around you by two-legged animals, if you can sometimes see the frightened kitten behind an executive's angry facade, then this book will really have done its job.

Finally, let me make two rather technical points about the writing of this book. First, I can never think of a pet as "it," so to avoid the continual use of "he or she" and "him or her," I have alternated the gender of pronouns that refer to unnamed animals from chapter to chapter.

Second, in this book I tell many stories of real people who came to my office for medical help for their pets when the cure for the problems was an alternative one. Those stories happened in the past, and I tell them in the past tense. However, to prevent confusion about what happened when, I have used the present tense to describe my veterinary office and the techniques I first used there. The purpose of this book is to focus on ideas, not to record a historically accurate account of their development.

In my practice I learned many of the rules of the amazing Pet Game, and I am constantly learning more. It's always a great moment when I see a pet thinking *Rats! This guy's on to me.* As you discover some of the secrets of the game and apply them in your life with your pet—or your boss—I expect you'll worry less, laugh more, see yourself better, and stop spending your life doing little tricks your pet—or some fellow human—has taught you.

—Herbert Tanzer, D.V.M.

I would like to thank all the people
I have interacted with during the past
fifteen years for their listening,
which I consider a great gift.

CHAPTER I

It Doesn't Work Here!

THE OLD COUPLE WERE TERRIFIED. They sat anxiously in my waiting room, and when their turn came, they brought in their tiny, adorable Yorkshire terrier named Irving. The Yorkie had wide, sad, frightened eyes—and a perfectly dreadful cough. The way they held the little dog close and stared at it showed me how frightened they were.

They had been to half a dozen veterinarians, they told me, and the problem had been positively diagnosed as a collapsed trachea. x-rays had supported this diagnosis, and they had been told that a tracheal implant—surgical insertion of a piece of plastic to widen the narrow area in the windpipe—was required. They had been referred to me, a Yorkie expert. They wanted my opinion of the case.

I looked at the little dog on the table. No animal ever looked so forlorn. Irving coughed and opened his eyes still wider, apparently suffering from the immense trauma of being at a doctor's office again.

A collapsed trachea, a constriction of the windpipe two-thirds of the way down into the chest, seems to be fairly common in the breed; veterinary literature reports that it definitely produces a cough. Irving had always coughed a little, but the cough suddenly got worse. When he started this new, rasping, choking noise, the couple took him to a doctor who advised medication. But the cough persisted. Then they took him to another vet, but the dog kept on hacking. Finally, after more doctors and some x-rays, they were told he needed surgery.

I looked at the concerned couple and then at the little dog on the table. He had a truly nasty cough. *Chuaugh. Chuaugh-chuaugh.* He gazed up at me piteously and seemed to say, *See how dreadfully sick I am. Chuaugh. Chuaugh. You're worried for me, too, aren't you, Doc? Chuaaaaugh. It's the end for me, isn't it?*

I asked the people when the cough had suddenly grown more severe.

"I don't really . . . remember," the man said.

I asked again, this time making it clear I wanted an exact answer.

"Listen to him, Faye!" the man said. "He wants me to remember *exactly.* How should I know? Three weeks. Maybe six weeks ago it got bad. Now it's worse and worse."

"Now, look," I said. "You've come to me for assistance, so play along with me. This detail happens to be important. I

know a specific date is hard to remember, but I know you
can remember it. Was it three or six weeks?"

Reassuring them that they could remember seemed to
help. "Faye," the man asked, "was it six weeks ago we came
back from the Adirondacks?"

"You know, come to think of it, Max, that's when it
started. It was the week we got back from the mountains. He
was so glad to see us. The cough got real bad then."

Suddenly, I started to laugh. The worried couple were
shocked. They were contemplating a colossal surgical procedure to rebuild Irving's windpipe, an operation that would
cost hundreds of dollars and actually put the dog's life in
jeopardy—and I was laughing! From their faces I could tell
what they were thinking: How come he's not so worried?

I stopped laughing but maintained an air of lightness as I
continued my line of questioning. "When does he cough
most?" I asked them.

"Mostly at night."

"When you're sleeping?"

"Always!"

I questioned them further and learned that they both
worked during the day; at night they went to bed early.

There it was, the last piece of the puzzle. I addressed the
couple. While they were at work, I explained, Irving had
been lying around the house all day, being a dog. How would
they feel if they lounged around the house for ten hours and
then went to bed? They admitted they probably wouldn't be
tired.

"Sure," I said. "Irving goes to bed with you, sleeps for an
hour or so, isn't tired, wakes up, looks over, sees you both

sleeping, and says to himself, *There's no one to play with.* His two favorite playmates are sleeping. He gets upset. He remembers the two weeks when you went on your Adirondack trip and left him behind, which he took as abandonment, and that memory gets him *really* upset."

From the dog's point of view, the couple were necessary for his emotional survival. Their absence, which was also symbolized by their sleeping, threatened his survival. He subconsciously recalled how in the past these two nice people had always noticed his coughing. And in an attempt to get their undivided attention, he resorted to a familiar pattern—he produced a cough. It was magic! Immediately the bedroom light went on, and he heard the woman say, "Max, that poor little darling is choking to death!"

> *From the dog's point of view, the couple were necessary for his emotional survival. Their absence, which was also symbolized by their sleeping, threatened this survival.*

Far out! the dog must have thought. *It still works! Now I remember. Whenever I cough, they cuddle me to pieces. That's it! Chuaugh! If I cough and keep coughing, they certainly won't leave me alone again!*

The concerned couple, by responding to Irving's cough, merely reassured him that coughing was indeed a good way to avoid being left alone again.

They looked at me, perplexed. "Do you mean," the man asked, "he's coughing like that to get attention? That's ridiculous."

"I'll let you in on a secret," I whispered, moving away from Irving, who was taking all this in. "When you went away, he got frightened. He does have a collapsed trachea, but he's using it. It was always there—so how come the cough only got bad when you returned from your vacation?"

They shrugged.

"He's playing the 'Coughing-Dog Game' with you."

Irving, who had been listening to us intently and getting no attention whatever, suddenly began to cough. *Chuaugh. Chuaugh-chuaugh.*

I picked up the tiny dog, turned him toward me, looked him square in the eye, and said with utmost seriousness, "It doesn't work here. It doesn't work here, Irving!"

The dog stopped coughing.

Then I turned him around so he faced his owners directly. *Chuaugh. Chuaugh.* It was a dreadful cough, a lethal-sounding cough, indeed.

Then I turned him toward me again. "It doesn't work here," I told him.

There was a small cough.

I repeated my statement.

This time there was silence.

I turned him to face his owners and he coughed; I turned him back toward me and he stopped.

A twinkle of recognition came into their eyes . . . They'd been conned—and now they knew it. They knew that Irving's cough was just a game.

As they watched, their mouths dropped. A twinkle of recognition came into their eyes. They looked at each other and smiled as if a great weight had been lifted from their shoulders. They'd been conned—and now they knew it. They knew that Irving's cough was just a game.

They left my office a little later. As they walked through the crowded waiting room, I watched the man hold the

Yorkie up close to his face, as I had done, and say, "It doesn't work here. Irving, it does not work here any more. Not one bit!"

It hasn't always been like this in my office. I haven't always been able to find such happy remedies. I used to be a conventional veterinarian with an orthodox approach to veterinary medicine.

When I went to the prestigious veterinary college at Cornell University forty-six years ago, I was the typical over-achiever. I was so competitive and so afraid of flunking out that I won all the school's awards for medicine, surgery, and bacteriology. During the summers after my junior and senior years, I worked for a veterinarian who allowed me to do a great deal of surgery, and by the end of my senior year, having performed some four hundred to five hundred operations, I was an ace at it. I graduated first in my class. I had an abiding belief in the truth of classical medicine. I chose a busy, urban practice and set out to become "Supervet."

Though my practice flourished and I did a good job, I began to doubt that much of what I did was really helping

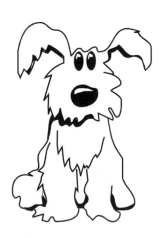

the pets. There was so much I didn't know. Why was there so much skin disease, which no one really understood? Some days I'd see twenty cases of dogs and cats mutilating themselves by licking or scratching. What caused so much itching? Why were certain diseases seasonal? I wasn't satisfied with what classical veterinary literature said caused these problems, so I started to look elsewhere. Since I was the most available animal for me to study (even though I walked on my hind legs most of the time), I decided to use myself as a research subject, and I looked to see what made me tick.

As my consciousness expanded, I became less limited by classical, scientific, rational ideas. I also sensed that I was affected by feelings of fear, pain, and anger that I had not fully experienced—that I had not allowed to run their course. Then the way I experienced the relationship between pets and their owners began to change dramatically. I became aware that I was totally responsible for everything in my life, and I realized that this was also true of pet owners. They, too, were responsible for what was happening in their lives, including the behavior of their pets.

Although my self-searching did not provide answers, it created an opening for me to *see* pet problems with more clarity and treat them in ways I think are more truthful—and fruitful.

One case in particular, which occurred during this evolution of mine, drove home to me the fact that conventional medicine did not seem to be the answer in quite a number of the cases I was treating. One day an elderly man came in with a dachshund who wasn't eating very well. The dog had been a voracious eater; he had been bouncy and enthusiastic whenever the owner came home or wanted to take him for a walk. Now he wasn't. By the owner's standards, the animal was hardly eating. And now the little dog calmly walked out of the house instead of jumping for joy at the sight of the leash.

I examined the dog. The results were negative—no organic problems.

Was it possible that the problem lay *outside* the animal? I'd been trained to think otherwise. All my specialized training had pointed me toward the organism, the pet's *body;* the problem *had* to be mechanical, one of "plumbing." But what if it wasn't? I began to look outside, to explore the animal's environment, to shift my focus from the animal himself to the total picture.

I asked the owner how long the dachshund had shown such symptoms.

"Oh, perhaps two or three weeks," he said. "And I feed him the same food."

No, it wasn't the food; that was the organic approach again—too reasonable, much too reasonable. That approach was the way I'd always thought about such problems, the way virtually all owners thought of them. I was looking for something else this time and had to free myself from all previous associations.

"Don't tell me about what you *think* is causing the problem," I said suddenly. "Tell me what's going on in *your* life."

He didn't know what I meant.

"Has anyone come to live with you?" I ventured. "Has anyone gone away? Did you get new drapes, a new rug? I'm groping, exploring. I'm not even sure what I'm looking for. Are you home more? Or less?"

"Surely," the man said, becoming rather stiff-lipped, "you don't want me to believe that any of *those* things are causing him to starve himself to death."

I told him the dog—who was perfectly healthy—was in no such danger but that I really didn't know what was causing the change in behavior. Yet as I thought about it, I realized that maybe, just possibly, such matters did serve as causes.

"Well, nothing's changed," he kept insisting until I learned, finally, that he had retired three weeks earlier and was now home almost all day, every day. The dog's new behavior had, by coincidence, started the day after the man retired.

Later that night I began to think about the case. I reasoned that the dachshund loved this old guy and that when the owner was at his job, the dog felt unhappy and threatened in some way, so he resorted to some classic Freudian patterns like overeating. When the owner came back home or wanted to go for a walk, the dog became so overjoyed he virtually shouted, *Hey, thank God you're back! I need you!*

Now he had the owner all the time. Now they went out together so often it was no longer an occasion for jumping up and down. Now the dog didn't have to overeat. In fact, he was being absolutely normal and contented and was saying, *It's terrific. I've got you all the time.* And he was so satisfied emotionally that he slept most of the day and ate much less.

That case opened an entirely new field to me. As owners brought me their pets, I began to explore each animal's environment, his *owner's* behavior patterns, and the nature of the games that went on between the two. I became, to my great fascination, a sleuth, probing into the *real* reasons for so many of the illnesses I'd never fully understood, ferreting out the real causes of kooky behavior in pets.

To treat the pet properly, I soon realized, I had to treat not merely the plumbing problem—which often *did* have to be treated clinically—but the whole situation that had created it. I realized also that there was some great drama, some larger game, taking place between human and animal, and I wanted to learn about it—discover its rules—so I could play my part in it wisely.

> *To treat the pet properly, I soon realized, I had to treat not merely the . . . problem . . . but the whole situation that had created it.*

A number of years have passed, and the game is clearer to me now. I have seen and treated thousands of cases in that time—some two hundred a week—with many startling results. My view of illness has changed dramatically. I hope I have allowed people to see more clearly where they stand in reference to their pets—which may also be where people stand with reference to themselves and their environment. This has made my work enormously satisfying.

CHAPTER 2

Doctoring

AFTER TWENTY-SOME YEARS OF PRACTICE, I found myself
with some gray hair, a doctor's jacket, a stethoscope, and the right
terminology on my tongue. I was a competent diagnostician. I knew
the names of all the animal diseases. I could administer all the standard treatments, but these days something else is possible—a
whole other approach to practice. The real contribution I have to
make lies in showing owners their animals' psychological nature.
Both pets and owners can best be served by helping the animals get
"unstuck" from the games they're playing and coaxing people not to
do things that get animals stuck in the first place in playing their
part in the game. Doctoring in such terms becomes a tremendously
creative experience.

If I were coaching a young veterinarian in this new approach to
"doctoring," however, I would warn him or her of certain pitfalls.

Many people are simply not ready to hear anything other than
what they expect from a doctor; it upsets them if they cannot

squeeze the doctor into their systems of belief. They want to hear a few Latin words they don't understand; they want to see the doctor use a hypodermic needle; they want to watch him or her scrawl out an undecipherable prescription. That makes the process reliable. They want the security they've been led to expect from doctors. And often that's the only way the doctor can appropriately serve them. Some people won't accept anything but a standard medical line from me. But I always try.

The real contribution I have to make lies in showing owners their animals' psychological nature. Both pets and owners can best be served by helping the animals get "unstuck" from the games they're playing and coaxing people not to do things that get animals stuck in the first place in playing their part in the game.

Always, before I do anything else, I examine the animal and discover precisely what—if anything—is wrong with her physically. After I finish my basic physical examination, my job becomes that of a detective. I need to trace the trail of evidence and learn what game is being played, by whom, and for whose benefit. There is only one way to do this—I need to get people to talk. And before they will talk, I need to create a "safe space" for the discussion. I hint that Whiskers might, just possibly, be playing a game. "Pets are potential Academy Award winners," I tell owners.

Humor often helps to loosen people up. In fact, if I can get the seriousness of the situation out of the way, I have a foot in the door. "If you really want something to worry about," I continue, "my secretary will give you our Worry

List. But believe me, this dog is a better actor than Kevin Costner."

In some cases this builds enough safe space. In other cases, owners are still leery.

"All right," I tell them. "I can play 'Real Doctor.' I can give Whiskers *real* medicine, *real* ointments, *real* pills, and *real* treatments for the *real* disease. We can even keep him in our *real* hospital for three days. The dog will be a *real* patient. You'll be a *real* nurse and concerned parent. The drug company will get to play 'Real Drug Company' with *real* drugs. Everybody wins! It's a terrific game. I even get *real* money. And you get a chance to come back and play again next week—and give me more *real* money."

I pause.

"Or we don't have to play it that way. We can do something else. Something that's fun, too. It may seem totally unreasonable to you. I know dozens of other veterinarians who will say I'm insane. It may even look as if I'm making myself unnecessary. For although your pet's disease is real, you simply may not need a doctor. There may be an alternative way of dealing with the disease."

Maybe it is the ridiculousness of the situation, the fact that they might save some money, the assurance that Whiskers is not physically ill, or mere curiosity—but if I can get to this point, I can usually begin my questioning.

Let me show you how this works, using what I call the "Case of the Twitching Beagle." A woman and her grown daughter brought in a beagle named Bagel with a pronounced muscular twitch involving his face, his shoulder, and the right side of his neck. The twitch looked bad. Each of the women was fifty pounds overweight, the dog a full ten. The three of them, nervously lined up together outside the exam room door, were so deadly serious that they looked like Rodin's *Three Shades*. The women were certain Bagel was at death's door.

As I examined the dog, the twitching began in earnest, and from the weary, sad look in his eyes, I knew he was thinking, *Oh, no. Look where they've brought me. It's all over. This is the end of old Bagel.*

I did not tell the dog *not* to be afraid; I allowed him to experience his initial fears while I gave him a thorough physical examination. By the time I was through, I could see that the fear had eased. But the twitch was even worse. It looked exactly like what I would once have treated as a neurological problem, the kind that usually occurs as a sequela to (aftereffect of) distemper. But I'd known this dog since he was a pup; he'd never displayed a single symptom of distemper.

One way to handle the case would have involved my sending the owners to a neurologist, which would have cost them four hundred to five hundred dollars. The doctor might have been able to name the disease, but it was more likely that he or she would have said, "Unfortunately . . . ahem, ahem . . . there's no known treatment for this, and we really don't know what causes it. It may get better. It may not. In my experience . . . ahem . . . it usually clears up by itself in six months. Or it may not."

What a marvelous game! Again, everybody got something. I got to be the guy smart enough to know he didn't know enough, who referred the patient to someone who did; somebody got to play neurologist; the dog got a chance to be

sick, with all the attention that usually comes from that state
of things; the owners got a chance to be the "Anxious Owners"; the neighbors got a chance to be "Concerned Neighbors." And everyone would be clinging to this game for dear
life.

Death's door, indeed!

I looked at Bagel, but not with a
grim professional visage. I was smiling
at him knowingly. His shoulder, neck,
and jaw muscles were *all* twitching
merrily away now, but the look in his
eye said, *The rat. The louse. He's going*

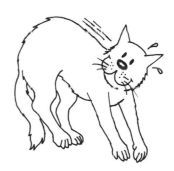

to give me away. Oh, I just know it. His manner was definitely
embarrassed. This was probably the first time since he'd
started to twitch that anyone had failed to take him seriously.
I'd seen the same embarrassment dozens of times before
when I was about to expose other pets as frauds.

I completed my examination. Bagel had no organic problems whatsoever. I chuckled, turned to the two women, and
said, "Listen. This dog is not going to die from this shaking.
It looks terrible. You think he's going to have a convulsion any
minute and drop dead. But it's not going to happen. He
doesn't have a serious disease. I promise. So let's enjoy this."

The women were immediately relieved. (For years I'd
thought my drugs were curing pets; instead, it was probably
my green jacket, stethoscope, diplomas on the wall, and
assurances that made owners unworried—and pets better.)
They were thinking, The doctor said it's all right, so it must
be all right. We don't have to worry. Bagel is not going to die.
It's a miracle.

I asked them when Bagel twitched most, and the mother said, "All the time. During the day. But especially at night, when I'm sleeping."

I asked her how she could possibly know he was twitching when she was asleep. It was not a silly question. Clearly, she woke up periodically during the night and with great concern, went to the dog—all because of that twitch! Her answer confirmed my suspicion.

"Now," I asked, "when did you see the twitching begin?" This was and is an interesting issue. Most people go blank when I ask them this question. They know that their dogs twitch or cough or whatever but not precisely when these symptoms started. The owners don't seem to want to be clear about what is really happening, to understand that their pets are not really sick. They inwardly want to maintain the game.

"I can't remember," Bagel's owner said.

I pressed her.

"Oh, I don't know . . . three, maybe four weeks ago. No. Maybe it was only two weeks ago."

"Was it two or three or four? Think carefully."

She couldn't remember.

"You can't remember two or three weeks ago?"

"I really can't," she said.

"If you *could* remember, when would it be?"

"Okay. Two weeks ago. Is this *really* important to Bagel's twitching, Dr. Tanzer?"

"What day was it?"

"How would I *possibly* know?"

I kept questioning and finally learned that the twitching had definitely begun two weeks earlier, on a Wednesday.

It was a start.

"Fine," I said. "Now what happened on Tuesday of that week?"

I could see that both women were becoming involved in the game, but neither could remember what had happened the day before the twitching began.

"Something happened," I insisted.

"Well," the daughter said, "we changed his food. Could that . . . "

"No. Not what happened in *his* life. I want to know what happened in *your* lives. What happened in the house? Did someone come to visit? Did someone go away? Perhaps you got a new chair."

"Well," the woman said, looking at me strangely, as if I were clairvoyant, "we did put a new slipcover on the chair in the living room."

"That's *his* chair, right?"

"Well . . .yes, it is."

"Fine. That's it."

They looked at me. "What do you mean, 'That's it'?"

By this time the two women were playing along. They were ready for the next step. But when pet owners aren't ready, I engage them by asking what they *think* is causing the disease. For example, in the case of an infected ear, I let the owner tell me, "I might have gotten water in the ear."

"All right."

"Or it might have been the flea shampoo I used last week."

"Anything else?"

"Well, my friend Sally thinks it could be ear mites."

I allow her to empty out, to flush away everything she thinks could be causing the problem—what she's read, what friends have told her, what her friend's veterinarian thinks. Then I say, "None of that is causing the infection. Would you agree, though, that if we can find the cause, we have a chance of curing this?"

"Certainly."

"Well, I know the cause."

She then looks at me in amazement.

"Let's see if I can show you what it is." And I begin a little game I have worked up.

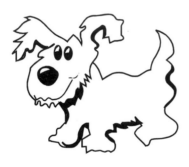

In the "Case of the Twitching Beagle," I began the game with the mother and daughter. To start, I told them, we needed players, a board to play on, a definition of winning, and a set of rules. I agreed to play that notorious Academy Award winner, Bagel; the mother agreed to play herself. Next I described the board we would play on. My office would be their house, my cabinet their television set, my chair Bagel's chair. "The rules are simple," I explained. "Every time I twitch, like this," and I mimicked Bagel's twitch in an exaggerated fashion, "you must come over and look at me and say, 'Oh, my poor baby. What's wrong with him, Florence?' Do you agree to do that?"

Both women laughed, and the mother agreed.

"My definition of winning the game," I said, "is getting you to come over and cuddle me. That's what I'm after. Got it?"

They said they did.

"Now, I'm Bagel. I really love you. I love you people like mad. I love it when you watch your television set and I curl up in my chair, like this." I sat in my office chair and rested my head and arms on the armrest. "I look over, and there you both are, and here I am in my chair, and it's delicious. Then, two weeks ago, on a Tuesday, I jumped up on my chair and suddenly heard, 'Get that damned dog off the chair! We just spent seventy dollars for that new slipcover.' So I got thrown off my chair, and boy, was I frightened! Again I jumped up on the chair, and again you shouted, 'Get off! It'll get dirty!' Then I really began to tremble, and when I noticed you two looking at me, I started to shake. Maybe the chair is just the beginning. Maybe you two are going to get rid of me. Maybe I don't count around here any more. And suddenly I realized that when I started to shake, you started to pay attention to me. So every time you threw me off the chair after that, I shook a little more—and it snowballed.

"You remember the rules we agreed on," I said to the women, "so let's pick up the game at that point."

I began to twitch violently, and the mother just sat there. "No, no, no," I said. "You agreed to play. I'm Bagel." I twitched again. This time, tentatively, shyly, she got up, then thought it was all too silly for words and sat down again. "You agreed," I insisted. This time I gave a momentous series of twitches and she came over, laughing, and began to say "poor-baby" to me. She wasn't a very good actress. I suspected she was much more convincing with Bagel. We repeated the routine several times. She laughed and then did it more readily.

"Great," I told her. "Shaking—that's surely the way to Mommy's heart. So I shake a little more, and you two get even more worried. You begin to *care* about me. Then I add a few very special variations. Boy, do they work! This *is* the right way to get attention. I may even go on and have a convulsion."

Then I stopped. I changed my tone. "If in fact this dog is shaking and twitching because he wants your attention and you are giving him attention because he's shaking, then who is causing him to shake?"

It was a touchy moment. Some people won't answer this question. One man said at this stage in his game, "You're making fun of me, Doctor, and I don't like it a bit." I gave him a bottle of pills to be taken by his cat three times a day for a disease that didn't exist. Another owner called me a quack. Some people just nod ambiguously.

The mother nodded.

"No," I said. "Tell me. In words. Who, precisely, is causing this?"

She gave another nod.

"Come on!"

"Okay, okay," the owner of the beagle finally said. "I am. I'm causing Bagel to shake."

"Wow!" I said. "Everything that's driving you crazy, the very thing you came in here for, *you're* causing. Isn't that a gas?"

At this point some people leave; others flay me with insults. It all takes time, and using this technique requires my spending many more hours with animals than I used to. But when their owners finally understand, I know I have truly served them. I might earn less money now, but I feel far more satisfaction.

I have used this method over and over. I love to see how the same old game varies, the dazzling number of different ways in which it's played.

One dog had a spur of calcium in its neck. This is a real medical problem. How had it snowballed into a severe spasm? Where did one cat's inflamed vulva come from? Why had another dog suddenly, in its middle years, started to urinate on the rug?

It is always a fascinating hunt. And when I can get someone to say and mean, "This dog is twitching and I'm causing it to twitch"—when people begin to accept themselves as the cause—the problem has already begun to disappear and I know I have really done something for the pet. But this process can be difficult. People do not want to be responsible. They want to blame their pet's condition on "that germ," "that food," or "ear mites," not on themselves.

Even more difficult is getting people to understand that they might be able to make their pets' diseases disappear. They caused these problems, and really only they can cure them. I bring the owners to a moment of choice: continue to play the game or end it. If they can't participate in the cure, I need to treat the case in classical fashion. But wherever there is a chance to show them what is really

> *Even more difficult is getting people to understand that they might be able to make their pets' diseases disappear. They caused these problems, and really only they can cure them.*

happening in their lives—and in their pets' lives—I feel obligated to try.

Bagel's owner agreed to stop paying attention when the dog twitched, so we used no medication. Several weeks later the owner reported that the dog was cured.

I told her Bagel was a game player and was probably at this moment planning to go into act 2, urinating on the corner of the rug.

"Oh," she said, "He's already doing that."

The cure doesn't always work. Some pets are simply getting too much benefit, in too many ways, from the game; they will literally die to win—and some do.

Some people do not understand or want to cooperate. But it is always sweet when the "cure" works. And sometimes the process even changes the owner's whole life—which is sweeter still.

CHAPTER 3

Creating the Games

WHAT, PRECISELY, ARE THESE GAMES I've mentioned? In what way do they begin, and how do they explain the interaction between pet and owner?

"Imagine a point on the surface of a sphere," I often tell owners, "and let that point represent your pet. The sphere is the pet's universe, and that point by itself is *nowhere* as long as the pet exists without significant context." Then you, an owner, come along and become—for whatever reasons—related to the animal. When you appear on the sphere too, your pet has a reference point. This dog or cat knows when he is in the world because he exists a certain distance and direction from you. He now feels he is *somewhere*. He has an experience of self, or identity, through your presence."

If the owner leaves the pet's sphere (goes on a trip or maybe just takes a nap) or perhaps changes his or her position on the sphere (becomes, for example, less interested in the pet), the pet no longer has a familiar reference point to relate to. He may in fact experience being *nowhere* again. That makes the pet worry about whether he will survive. A pet who feels his survival is threatened will usually resort to whatever game will work to ensure that the owner will remain *there,* close by, on the sphere. Nobody—human or animal—wants to be *nowhere.*

Even small changes in the owner-pet relationship can seem threatening to the pet. Owners think some threats are so slight that they roar with laughter when I suggest that the act of replacing Poopsie's favorite rug and refusing him access to the new one can cause bizarre behavior patterns, even disease. But it can.

What will the dog or cat do to keep his owner *there,* to re-establish his place on the sphere? There is a simple, one-word answer: *anything.* A pet quickly learns that one of the most effective ploys is developing a nice, showy malady: a very convincing cough, a twitch, diarrhea, skin lesions, a dietary problem, an eye disease, or any other illness. The range is quite extraordinary in the "Sick-Pet Game." The pet's action may be frightening or painful, but at least the pet knows he exists somewhere.

The pet's game is only half the story. The owner plays a role in the game and the two roles always correspond.

Let's go back to our sphere, and this time let the sphere represent the *owner's* universe. Create a point on the surface of that sphere and let that point represent the owner. That point by itself is nowhere; it too exists without significant context. When the pet appears on the sphere, the owner, like the pet, now has an additional reference point. He or she exists at a certain distance and in a certain direction from the pet. The owner now has a feeling of self, or identity, through his or her relationship to the dog or cat. As you can see, the owner-pet relationship is entirely reciprocal; it works both ways.

If the pet becomes ill, other characters, such as veterinarians, nurses, or attendants, take positions on the sphere. These characters on the sphere intensify the owner's experience of being *somewhere*. In other words, we complicate our lives because we want to feel we are somewhere. The more entangled our existence, the more difficult it is to untangle. The tangle provides safety. After all, if our entanglements persist and we are part of them, then surely we will survive.

> *Owners are the central players in the Sick-Pet Game. Whether they know the difference between loving their pets and what I call caring for them may well determine the outcome of the game.*

Owners are the central players in the Sick-Pet Game. Whether they know the difference between *loving* their pets and what I call *caring* for them may well determine the outcome of the game. Caring is what owners have been programmed to believe they must do for their pets. "Of course I care!" they say indignantly. The dog is coughing or twitching or licking or urinating in the house, and they *know* that what they're supposed to do is *care* about this. They also begin to worry, which is a real waste of time.

The owners fret over the alarming symptoms and care; in short, they give the pet *attention,* which means the pet has won the Sick-Pet Game. The pet perceives that his cough or twitch is indeed the way to maintain—or even improve—his position in the household, his position on the sphere. In fact, many pets see that they can actually run the household. Caring only perpetuates the game.

On the other hand, if the owners stop resisting, stop caring, the sickness may well disappear. *Loving,* a term I define as the antithesis of caring, is permitting a pet to be what he is, which may include being sick. This permission allows the game to stop temporarily. After all, the game requires the owner's active participation to continue. *Loving* the pet is simply letting him *be,* so he can finish being sick. Think of how you feel when you've been permitted to complete a piece of work on your own, putting together a bookcase or a quilt or a poem. When you complete the task, it disappears from your thoughts. When you complete a feeling or any experience, it too disappears.

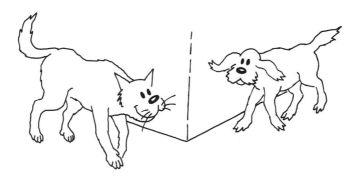

If you allow a pet to play out his drama, he can get on with and *complete* the experience of being sick and proceed to the experience of being healthy.

My proper role in such a game is to allow people to step out of the drama for a few moments—or forever—to look at themselves and their pets, to see how both are acting, and perhaps to understand why. But I can do relatively little until owners begin to understand that they have actually *created* their pets.

> Loving, *a term I define as the antithesis of caring, is permitting a pet to be what he is, which may include being sick.*

CHAPTER 4

Creating
Pets

THE IDEA THAT PEOPLE CREATE THEIR PETS is difficult to explain and even harder for many people to believe. It infuriates some and tickles others.

You'll have less trouble accepting the idea if you've noticed that a remarkable number of owners closely resemble their pets in their prominent physical characteristics. Over and over again I have seen people with long noses and lean bodies leading Doberman pinschers; small, short-legged people with pugs; elegant people with Siamese cats; and placid, easygoing people with sweet old tomcats. Watch pet owners and their pets on the street and I'm sure you too will see that some people unwittingly duplicate themselves in their pets. They are asking the world to agree that they are okay the way they are; if the world accepts their pets, it will accept them, too.

But others want pets that represent what they *would like to be*, pets that embody what the owners feel are more attractive or impressive characteristics than they themselves possess.

I had a weightlifter as a client. He was so short I could look down on him, and I'm not tall. He was almost as wide as he was high; his arms looked like my thighs, and I played defensive guard on Cornell's football team. He was a perfect brute of a human being.

The weightlifter's first dog was an Irish wolfhound, one of the tallest breeds of dogs. This particular creature was a towering specimen. When he stood on his hind legs, I had to stand on tiptoe to look at him properly. It was clear to me that despite the weightlifter's great bulk, he viewed himself as a tiny person and had re-created himself as this immensely tall dog. So emotionally tied was the man to the dog that he practically drove me crazy with extravagant concern over the wolfhound's health. If the dog got a splinter, the man insisted I take the animal into my hospital. Neither of them, man or dog, was ever, to my knowledge, really sick.

And then the dog was stolen or ran off.

The man was despondent for weeks. Finally, he called to tell me that he was flying from New York to the West Coast that night to pick up a new dog; he had to have the pet right away. His voice was urgent, as if this were a question of his survival. He wanted to know if I would be in the office the next day, a Sunday, so he could bring in the wolfhound's replacement. It was an Akita, a 160-pound Japanese dog

developed for guard work and hunting wolves, a veritable
monster.

I had seen far too many cases of the extraordinary identification of owners and their dogs to have the slightest shred
of doubt that this was just a coincidence.

Why did Telly Savalas have a bull mastiff who was ugly
to the point of being beautiful?

Was Falla, that nice, happy, little Scottish terrier, a coincidence at Franklin Roosevelt's comfy, cozy fireside chats?

Was Bill Sikes's brutish bulldog in *Oliver Twist* the result
of a chance decision by Charles Dickens?

Why did Lyndon Johnson pick up his beagles by the ears
for the cameras on the White House lawn? Was he revealing
his notion of his own power or perhaps indirectly demon-
strating that big-eared people can take it?

And what about Checkers, President Nixon's poor, forlorn cocker spaniel? He was just like poor Dick Nixon—
taken advantage of. Was this a coincidence?

Why, precisely, do people create their pets? Clearly, it is
to play out a drama in their lives that is not yet completed.
The bald man who came into my office with clenched teeth
and demanded that I tell him what to do about his collie's
"crazy shedding" had not yet accepted his own baldness. I
looked at the man's glistening scalp, listened to the tone of
his voice, and knew how much
he resisted hair loss. Only when
he could say, "It's all right for the
animal to lose its hair," would his
animal stop the excessive shedding and this particular drama be

> *Why, precisely, do people
> create their pets? Clearly,
> it is to play out a drama in
> their lives that is not yet
> completed.*

finished for him; only then would the man truly be free to get any kind of dog he wanted.

Is this theory unreasonable? Absolutely. These behaviors are based on unreasonable, alternative ways of thinking.

In terror, older people bring in aging but perfectly healthy pets they think are dying. One attractive elderly couple brought me their venerable tabby, who'd had a tumor removed from his mouth. The mouth had healed beautifully, but they were still frightened.

What are they doing here? I asked myself. Their anxiety is totally disproportionate to the reality of this situation, and they don't have an extra twenty-five dollars for this visit. What are they buying for this money and fear?

Then I realized that the cat was simply getting old and that they were experiencing their own old age, infirmities, and impending death through him. These realities were too difficult for them to face directly in themselves.

"Listen, you guys," I told them. "This cat is getting to be an *alter kaker* ("old geezer"). That's all. So he doesn't run up the stairs so quickly. Neither do you. It's all right to walk up slowly. There's nothing wrong with getting old. It's part of living."

Their faces lit up. They smiled. I'd given them license to get old. Most of the world says old age is not okay, and most older owners would put their old cats on Medicare if they could.

"Something else," I said. "He's going to die—no question about it—but not yet. He's still having a ball. Do you think he sits around worrying that he can't rush up the stairs? He goes up slowly, but he gets there anyway. He's enjoying his aliveness. Don't spoil it for him. There's no need to worry about death; it will find him. Pay attention to him now, and enjoy what life he has left."

As they walked out smiling, I realized that this was the best contribution I could make to their lives and to their tabby—helping them accept that growing old is all right. For their twenty-five dollars they had bought assurance that it's okay to age.

Some owners are chronic nurses and *must* adopt every stray cat or dog they find. I used to look in amazement at all the sick, repulsive, smelly cats that some people would regularly adopt out of the sewers and bring in. How could anyone pick up and fondle such creatures? I wondered.

One multimillionaire who rode around the city in a chauffeur-driven Cadillac could not resist such feline waifs and was forever having his driver stop in the middle of traffic to pluck a new one out of the gutter; then he'd drive the animal directly to my office. "Fix him," the man would say. "Do everything necessary to make him well and healthy, and then I'll take him home." He's done this *fifty* times in twenty years.

It happens that this client experienced what seemed like emotional abandonment when he was a child. Perhaps many other chronic adopters of abandoned, starving, or sick cats and dogs recall some comparable experience in their own lives that they haven't been able to accept. My questioning of such people leads me to believe this theory: When people feel abandoned or sickly, when they haven't completed and come to terms with their experiences, they adopt an animal to re-create their own dramas. The abandoned animal is a re-creation of themselves. In other words, they symbolically try to cope with their abandonment by adopting *themselves*. In fact, they *resist* completion (closure of their experience) by the very process of picking up every stray cat, and actually perpetuate the drama. One cat is some help to them but not enough. They happen, by coincidence, to find another. The second cat makes them feel even better but still not complete, so they adopt another and another. Finally they have thirty or forty cats and there's no end in sight. People clearly have to keep reliving the past until they have completed it. After that the past can be ignored or forgotten.

The game seems less serious when it's played with pets rather than people. The stakes aren't as high, and therefore the losses won't be as great if things don't work out.

Not long ago one forty-five-year-old unmarried woman, who has been coming to me for some years, entered my office crying her heart out. Whitey, a dog she loves deeply, had suddenly turned nasty.

"I love him, Dr. Tanzer," Marilyn said, her voice quavering, "but he bites me and snarls and is always mean now. I'm terrified of him, and I'm afraid to leave him alone with my mother in the house."

I was having a busy day, but I knew I had to give this woman some time. As I questioned her about Whitey, her home, and her aged mother, trying to see clearly what the drama was, I suddenly realized that the problem really lay in her relationship with her mother. The old woman was grumpy, nasty, even hostile. Marilyn loved her mother but hated living in the house with her. Unable to confront the real drama, she created a smaller, identical problem with her dog. She loved the dog but now either had to accept him the way he was, which was difficult, or get rid of him because of his hostility. Her anxiety lay in the fact that she had to make a choice but could not do it.

How could I help? I wondered.

"I want to tell you about my friend Charlie," I said. "He's one of the nicest guys I know. He's married and has two kids and a really pleasant house in the country. The only problem is that his mother lives with them, and she's a grumpy old witch who could easily make his life miserable. Ten times a week I ask him how he can put up with her. But the strange thing is that Charlie isn't miserable. He looks at the situation and says, 'She's my mother, and she's a grumpy old witch. But I'm going to live with her.' Charlie has *chosen* to live with this person. It may be scary—it may even be uncomfortable—but that's what you have to do with Whitey. *Choose* whether you want to live with Whitey or get rid of him. If you choose to keep him, you'll have to say, 'I'm going to live with this nasty old dog. I love Whitey, and I'll have to learn to handle being afraid.'"

What happened next might seem surprising. As soon as Marilyn chose to keep the dog—and changed her attitude—

> *Nothing about pets is ever a coincidence. The re-creations people produce with their pets sometimes become uncannily like the original situation.*

Whitey stopped getting negative signals from Marilyn and so stopped being nasty. I hoped I'd helped her with her deeper problem as well.

Nothing about pets is *ever* a coincidence.

The re-creations people produce with their pets sometimes become uncannily like the original situation. Miss
Holt, a thirty-eight-year-old single woman who had loved her
late father deeply and taken care of him for many years
before he died, had a ten-year-old male terrier who ran her
life with his sicknesses. I removed the dog's left testicle,
which had a tumor. Curiously, her father also had his left testicle removed because of a malignancy.

I treated one dog with a breast tumor. I removed it; it
returned. I removed it again; it returned again. I couldn't
understand. Then I learned that the owner's mother had
recently died from breast cancer.

When one dog I treated was upset, he would make the
sound *Whoooo, whoooo.* I'd heard the woman who brought
him in do the same thing. Her husband hated this sound and
hated when his wife did it, but he only said "Shut your trap"
to the *dog* because it was not all right for him to say this to
his wife.

Pets are safer.

I have a friend who has never completed a sense of sadness and abandonment (confronted and dealt with her feelings). She avoided letting those feelings spill over into her
interactions with her children, but she was often hysterical
and fearful about her dog because dogs are okay to be frantic
about. The children were happy and well adjusted; the dog
got sick every other week.

When one family was having marital problems, the family dog suddenly started a pattern of defecating on the rug.
The woman, who was wondering whether she really wanted
to stay married to her husband, kept saying, "You know, we

may have to get rid of that dog." To her the dog *was* her husband in this re-creation of the family drama. But when the problem cleared up for the human beings, it cleared up for the dog, too—and the woman couldn't imagine how she'd ever wanted to give up the dog.

To care for a pet, my medical training was not enough. Sometimes I had to understand the family situation as well, so that I could discover the origin of the pet's problems. It was important for me to learn as accurately as possible who the pet was and why it had been created.

One day an Irishman in his mid-forties—a tough guy with a face like putty and a red, bulbous nose—came in with a disgusted look and a fairly young Alaskan malamute. The owner had hair all over his face from the dog's intense shedding. The man's last dog had been a trim, well-trained German shepherd named Gray Fox, who would do anything his owner wanted. The shepherd had been *his* dog, not his wife's. The Alaskan malamute, Doris, was an unruly, hairy nuisance, whom I had been treating for three months for a series of skin diseases. The shepherd used to jump onto my examining table at the owner's command, but Doris refused repeated commands and merely wanted to be picked up. As the man wearily did so, he said, "This dog is such a pain. I need her like a hole in the head." He told me confidentially that when he got into bed with his wife at night, Doris got between them and literally pushed his wife out. I laughed and encouraged him to tell me more.

"This damned dog loves me," he said. "If I stop on the corner to rap with some male friends, everything's fine; but when I talk to a woman, Doris goes crazy, barking and carrying on so much I have to leave. And if I sit down on a couch and a woman friend of mine happens to sit next to me, watch out. The dog gets between the two of us and pushes her off with her feet. You'd almost think the dog was jealous."

I happened to know that the man had one particular female friend, with whom he did much more than sit on a couch—every Thursday night.

He went on and on and I couldn't help asking. "Who got this animal?"

"*I* got her." he said.

"*You* did?" She didn't sound like *his* dog.

"Yeah. On a Sunday. The day Gray Fox died my wife insisted we go right out and get another dog."

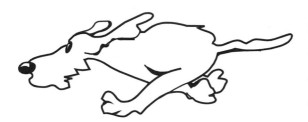

So that was it. His *wife* had created this hairy creature to serve as a guard. She knew about the Thursday-night woman friend and wanted to make sure there were no others. And crazy Doris loved the man to distraction, may even have felt married to him, and pushed away all women—including the wife who had created her!

One couple came in with an especially nasty German shepherd who ran their lives. I knew the man had a weak streak. The woman, however, was strong; she supported her mother, who came to dinner every Friday night. How that man suffered! I'd watched him for years. I could see how much quiet, restrained rebellion—even hostility—was inside him, though he rarely said a word.

Their dog didn't fool me, and despite their warnings that he was positively dangerous, I grabbed him by the lower jaw, told him I wanted no games, took a blood sample, and examined him at will.

The woman was amazed that I could get away with so much. "Look," she said, "what are we going to do with Bruno? He needs a psychiatrist. In the house he bites people, he chases them, and he barks like mad. It's terrible. Really."

I was in a jaunty mood after taming this brute so handily, so I said to her, "Isn't he exactly what you want? Your house is your fortress. In your house you want people to leave you alone. Right?"

"No."

"He's exactly what you want," I insisted.

"Absolutely not!"

"Come on. Be a sport. Admit it."

At which point the man butted in and said, "He's exactly what *I* want!"

I looked at him, startled. He had always been such a quiet and restrained man—and he was proving my diagnosis wrong.

"This dog knocked my mother-in-law on her ass last week," he said loudly. Then even louder he said, "I've wanted to do that for twenty years!"

I roared with laughter and finally said, "There are a few people I know who I think should be knocked down. Can I borrow him?"

If people have actually created their pets, it is possible to see the people themselves—who they are, what they're feeling—in the animals. In a curious way, I can "undress" many owners and sometimes be of genuine help to them in their lives, enabling them to see themselves in the curious mirror that is their pets.

One young woman who began to understand the disasters in her life through this technique told me, "I'd better get my life in order before I have a baby!" If she was causing her pet's problem, she realized, perhaps she was unconsciously causing *all* her other problems as well. The Sick-Pet Game had been an *opportunity,* not a disaster, for her. Someday she'll be a better mother because of what she learned about herself with her pet.

A frightened young woman in her mid-twenties has been coming to my office for years with various pets. Recently she came in with her cat. I immediately tried, as I always do, to establish eye contact with the animal, but I could not. The cat squirmed all over the table, always avoiding my eyes. I 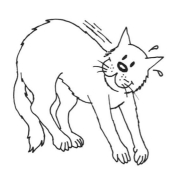 wanted to slip my hand under the cat's chin and get her to look directly at me. I wanted to tell her, "Look. Everything's all right. I'm not going to hurt you." Before I could do so, the cat jumped off the table and wriggled under a cabinet. When I tried to get at her, she hissed and extended a paw to scratch me but didn't seem to really want to. When I was finally able to make eye contact with the animal, I saw a softening take place in her face, and we went ahead with the examination with no problem.

Afterward, since I knew this young woman quite well, I took her into my office, where it was quiet, and talked for a few moments about my general concept of people creating their pets. She seemed receptive, so I said, "You know, that cat is a total re-creation of you."

She looked startled, as if she'd been found out. Then she looked away.

I described the animal's actions in some detail and saw that the woman was becoming more and more interested. I told her the cat did what she did. The cat avoided looking clearly at situations, and I suspected she did as well. Like the cat, she would run or become hostile if cornered.

She was looking away from me but turned back when I had finished. Our eyes met. "Dr. Tanzer," she said softly, "It's spooky being with you."

CHAPTER 5

The Acknowledgment Game

SOME PEOPLE CREATE A PET for acknowledgment.

Each year one breed or another seems to be in style, so an owner can feel important by creating a pet of that breed. Such people deliberately choose—or think they are choosing—an especially fine specimen. People who do this often doubt that they themselves are good specimens.

Let me make a composite portrait of a dozen men I've had in my office over the years with their "perfect" specimens.

I'll call this composite Sam. He is someone looking for something to do. He is successful but dissatisfied with his life. He buys a

$75,000 Mercedes, but he soon learns that he can't drive the car all day. Also, too many other people in his neighborhood own similar cars. He needs something else to prove he's important, prestigious. So he buys an enormous, beautifully built house. But he can't be in the house all the time either. He loses interest in it as soon as he's made all the adjustments and additions to the basic structure that he deems essential for a man of his stature. The house suits him—but it's not enough.

So Sam becomes interested in airplanes. He buys a twin-engine plane, becomes a great pilot, flies cross-country, and nearly dies in a crash. His survival further proves how great he is.

Finally, Sam reads in the newspaper about a dog show. He hears about pedigrees and championships for the first time.

"Ha," says Sam. "Never went to one of those. Bet the kids would love it."

He goes to a dog show, and as he looks at all the people and magnificent dogs on the field, he suddenly becomes intensely interested. A new game is starting for him.

It's all very "etiquetty." Each dog has a handler. Stern judges walk around the beautifully groomed and carefully posed dogs. When blue ribbons are presented, there is polite, meaningful applause. Sam watches in surprise as a woman walks over to one of the dogs, picks up his tail, and observes whether both the dog's testicles are there. The audience applauds when it's clear he's got both and is not disqualified.

This is *terrific,* thinks Sam.

"The winner," someone with a refined English accent announces, "is Sir Harry Royal Choice." There is more applause. Then the owner—Sam is already beginning to see himself as such an owner—comes out into the ring and receives a silver plate and there is more applause. What *acknowledgment!* Sam thinks.

"Maybe," Sam says that night on the way home, "we'll get ourselves a little dog."

The next day he sends his secretary to the library to find him pictures of all the classiest dogs. She brings back books with a dozen photographs marked. He lays them out on his desk and scrutinizes them. When he learns that the Bedlington terrier is particularly choice and rare—which will make Sam seem truly special—he decides on the spot. He *must* have a Bedlington terrier.

He makes phone calls and more phone calls until half the morning vanishes. The best kennels are in Toronto. He calls Toronto and makes an appointment to be there on Thursday. This couldn't be better, he thinks.

On Thursday morning Sam drives his Mercedes to the airport, gets into his $200,000 twin-engine plane, and zips confidently up to Toronto. At the kennel he is shown around by a pedigreed lady in tweeds and soon spots precisely the Bedlington terrier pup he *must* have—a champion if he ever saw one. Sam feels knowledgeable because he's read all about winners by now. In fact, he's read only three chapters in a book and two magazine articles. But the owner really hadn't intended to sell this particular pup, she says, because this one is special.

Immediately this pup becomes the one Sam surely has to buy.

No, the breeder insists, this one is simply not for sale. She's going to keep this one to show herself.

Finally, in what he thinks of as a colossal coup, Sam gets his dog. What a terrific animal. What a splendid woman to give it up, he thinks as he flies him home. He brings the dog into the house and announces, "Look, kids. We bought a little dog."

In fact, Sam hasn't bought a dog; he's merely made up a little toy for himself called the Dog. As part of his particular fight for survival, he's started another game, the "Perfect-Champion-Show-Dog Game." Despite all other appearances, he hasn't selected this dog—he's created him.

> *In fact, Sam hasn't . . . selected this dog—he's created him.*

A few days later, to make sure his dog is indeed a perfect specimen, Sam brings the Bedlington terrier to me. After examining the gorgeous animal for precisely thirty seconds and without any particularly elaborate diagnostic skills, I discover that Little Sir Royal Sam-Bed has an undescended testicle.

Sam is horrified. His face collapses. He sends his children out of the room. He says in a hoarse whisper, "Don't tell anyone about this, Doc."

"It's nothing that affects his health," I assure the anxious man. "You can't show him or breed him, but he'll make a lovely pet."

Lovely pet! thinks Sam. I have been duped.

"That woman in Toronto sold me an imperfect dog!" he shouts. He has re-created himself as a sexually defective dog. "It's horrible," he tells me. "Humiliating! There will be lawsuits. You must put this in writing."

In order for Sam to play the "I'll-Get-Back-at-That-Woman Game," I must immediately draw up a document that declares, "I certify that Sam's dog has only one testicle."

Actually, if Sam had been wise enough, he'd have seen that this situation was a chance for him to think about his own feelings of sexual inadequacy and make them unimportant.

But let's switch scenes in this composite picture of a dog owner and choose another ending to the scenario. Let's say I discover that the dog is indeed perfectly developed and healthy.

Sam now puts out his chest, nods knowingly to his children, and says, "Great, I knew it. I could see he was a champion the moment I saw him. I have an eye for champions. I told you, didn't I, kids?"

Now Sam really gets to work on the new project. He hires a handler. The dog's hair is sculpted impeccably, and his nails are trimmed. The dog is taught how to walk and how to put his tail up to exhibit to the world that he has two testicles.

And Little Sir Royal Sam-Bed, after thousands of dollars of training and upkeep, is indeed a champion. He's so successful that in time his reproductive potential is extremely valuable. People will now have to pay to have Sam's dog's semen, and Sam can be selective about whose dog he lets his dog mate with. The dog brings him praise, money, and sex appeal, the ultimate acknowledgment.

Is this success, finally, enough?

Not for a man like Sam.

There are those that feel life is a game. If this is true it follows that without a game, there is no life.

One day he calmly announces, "I'm thinking of buying a little horse for my daughter. I saw a rather reasonable Welsh pony for only $27,000."

And he goes on to the "Horse-Show Game," with all its struggles and victories!

There are those that feel life is a game. If this is true, it follows that without a game, there is no life.

Is it any wonder Shakespeare wrote that life "is a tale, told by an idiot, full of sound and fury, signifying nothing."

CHAPTER 6

In the Office

IN THE OLD DAYS, when I was a conventional veterinarian, I handled animals in the conventional way. If the animal wouldn't cooperate promptly, I had it muzzled and restrained. Particularly troublesome pets were anesthetized either with a hypodermic needle or with a dart containing a sedative. But that kind of treatment created more problems than it solved. A pet handled like a wild animal may, in fear, defecate, urinate, or empty its malodorous anal sacs; it may be harmed physically or harm someone in the room. In addition, pets who have suffered such treatment at the hands of one veterinarian and then go to another will take one whiff, smell danger, and begin the whole sordid scene again.

As I began to learn more about suppressed feelings, I saw more and more examples of this same fear among the people who came to my office. One owner came in with his little boy and a dog. The boy was petrified when I put the dog on the table. He was shivering and withdrawn, almost crying, and I heard his father say, "Don't be afraid, Billy."

Why not? Why shouldn't he be afraid? The man was teaching his own son that it was wrong to be afraid, and I suddenly realized that if he allowed the boy to experience the feeling, to be as afraid as he had to be, the fear might well vanish. When you experience an emotion to completion, it loses its hold over you.

The same holds true for pets. When I first realized this fact, I began groping for some way of entering the pets' world quickly and unthreateningly, some way to let them know I understand their fears. But I had no idea how.

One morning an owner brought in a big, ferocious dog. Veterinarians these days see a lot of dogs like this, bought by people who either are afraid of muggers and burglars or who are trying to pass themselves off as formidable. As cantankerous as this dog appeared, snarling and baring her fangs and straining at the leash, I found myself hating the idea of muzzling her and going through the whole dangerous and disagreeable routine for handling frightened animals. Instead, I sat down on the floor in front of the dog and instinctively opened my legs.

The dog seemed startled.

"Hey," I told her gently, "I know it's tough having all these giants walking around on their hind legs towering over you. But I'm down here. I'm on your level now."

My position, with legs spread and genital area unprotected, was open and vulnerable, a position dogs take when they want to show one another that their intentions are peaceable. I took the dog's leash and steadily, firmly, pulled her over to stand between my legs, so that with one move she could have made my voice rise nine octaves.

The dog looked at me, snarled slightly, and seemed to wonder, *What the heck is this guy doing? I'd better bite him. No. I really don't want to. Strange. Never saw this before.*

I felt her relax as she stood between my legs. With my position I'd said, "That's how much I trust you." And because I trusted her so much, she knew she could trust me.

Talking to her constantly, I had someone hand me in turn the two syringes I needed. Without using an ounce of restraint, allowing the dog to be afraid if that's what she wanted to be, I injected her twice. The dog scarcely twitched when the needles were inserted.

Then when I let her go, she rushed back to her owner and snarled and became "Hostile Dog" again.

I have had a few animals I could not immediately handle—but not too many. One angry, frightened man brought in his angry, frightened 120-pound German shepherd, Jacko. The games the dog was caught up in were bad ones; he'd bitten his owner and seemed quite eager to take a chunk out of me.

I knew at once that I could not handle this furious dog, so I asked the owner to leave him with me at the hospital for the day. I needed time. I wanted to create a relationship with this dog, and I knew I could not do so quickly.

I tied the dog to a cabinet in a busy part of the hospital, right in the middle of the room. For several hours, every time I walked by I'd try to stand still for a moment and just be there—my mind empty and clear—with the dog. He'd growl. *Grrrrrr. Rurrrrrrh!* Then he'd snarl a little and show his teeth.

I'd just acknowledge tacitly that he was terrified and therefore angry. I let Jacko see that he was safe with me. By not
resisting his hostility, I was making it possible for that hostility to vanish. That is, when he was afraid and I understood
and felt his fear in me, Jacko became less afraid. When I
re-created the feeling in me, I erased it in him. It took three
hours for him to experience all the fears he had concerning
veterinarians, but at the end of that time the dog was empty
of considerations and I was able to examine him without
incident.

Complications often arise through the owner's actions.
One owner will put his pet on the table and be afraid
because his animal is afraid. He's
also afraid that I am not going to
like *him* because his animal looks
so hostile. The owner's desperate
attempts to calm the animal only
make her *more* frightened. Saying
"It's okay. Don't be afraid" only
encourages the dog to resist her
fears. And if the dog resists the
experience of that fear, she does
not let it go to completion; thus,
she can't get over it. Hence the fear persists. In such cases I
must insist that the owner be silent.

"What do you do that's different?" a man who had been a
dog trainer for twenty years once asked me. "Whenever I
bring my dog in, I watch you. I've never seen pets react to a
veterinarian the way they react to you. Do you hypnotize
them?"

*Complications often arise
through the owner's
actions. One owner will
put his pet on the table
and be afraid because his
animal is afraid . . . The
owner's desperate attempts
to calm the animal only
make her* more *frightened.*

No, I don't hypnotize them.

I told the man as truthfully as I could that I *communicate* with them. "I *get* what they put out, and something comes out of me that *they* get. I talk to them, but the communication isn't verbal. I think I convey safety. That's chiefly what I try to do. They know I'm not going to hurt them—and that I see through their games."

I always try to establish immediate eye contact. I relax my eyes and try to convey my intentions and feelings; sometimes I must take a dog's chin or head in my hand and draw her eyes to mine. I am aware that not my words but the sound of my voice is important, but I use the right words anyway, words that carry my meaning. I try to listen to the animals, to hear what they are saying.

For example, take Wolf. *Arrrh grr. Arrrh ahh,* he says.

What is the dog telling me? I ask myself.

He snaps at me but misses; he doesn't really want to bite me, but feels obliged to try since he's been trained to think he is mean. *Arrrh-arr.* The sound is softer.

I don't resist. "I understand that you don't like this," I say. "But it's got to be done. I know you're afraid and that's perfectly all right in here. We're not prejudiced against scared dogs. It's not my intention to cause you pain, but there may be a little."

The dog makes a few, much quieter, sounds.

I ask, "Finished now? Ready to get on with it?"

He is. So I pick him up, put him on the table, and do what I have to do.

Once the pet and I reach an agreement, there is usually no trouble during the examination—unless the owner pipes up with, "Don't be afraid, Wolf." This immediately breaks the spell. Wolf then goes back to resisting his fear, and the fear naturally persists.

Sometimes, with a series of particularly vicious dogs, I feel as if I have armor on and I could tame lions! At other times, when I am preoccupied, this method doesn't work; I've had mornings when I've been bitten, nicked, or scratched by just about every cat and dog I saw. It becomes frightening. Then I go into my private office and ask myself, "What am I doing today? Where am I?" I sit down for fifteen minutes and observe my thoughts so I can truly *be* with the animals.

The office itself becomes a board in the "Pet Game." The dogs come to play their games—"Sick Dog," "Ferocious Dog," "Friendly Dog"—and the people come to play their games, too.

When I watch people encounter my receptionist, I see clearly that life is a continuum of game playing. Pet owners come to play the Sick-Pet Game with Dr. Tanzer, and they are promptly confronted by a barrier, my receptionist, who stands between them and playing the game they have come to play. Automatically owners shift gears and flow smoothly into the new game of removing the barrier that confronts them. The new game, called "Destroy-the-Receptionist Game," is a fun game in itself; it often occupies owners until they get to play the game in the main arena, my exam room.

I have always instructed my secretaries to provide an air of certainty in the waiting room, to assure people that everything possible is being done to prevent a long wait, and to make it clear that they are being seen in proper turn. My receptionist acknowledges the owners' presence and, if necessary, the fact that we are late, wrong, evil, impossible. This technique immediately short-circuits the Destroy-the-Receptionist Game and allows her to direct the owner to the "Waiting-Room Game," which itself is often full of anxiety, hostility, or even pleasure. Some owners enjoy it so much out there in the waiting room that they become immersed watching the other dogs and owners and don't really want to leave and come in to play the Sick-Pet Game.

Some people become so caught up in the office games that I see them with exceptional frequency. When I have to tell them the game is over—Poopsie has only a minor benign cyst, not a terminal tumor—they are positively upset; their faces collapse. I never worry, though; they are usually the kind of people who find something else to worry about soon enough.

Some owners positively need the drama of the office. Mrs. Tannenbaum, for instance, is pathologically unable to wait outside in the waiting room. Every visit is urgent. She has to come in immediately to disclose the terrible diseases her dogs are dying from. She herself has been actively dying for fifty years.

Mrs. Tannenbaum recently hobbled in briskly, out of turn, with her tiny, toothless Chihuahua. Her voice was rapid, high-pitched, and raspy as usual.

> *Some people become so caught up in the office games that . . . when I have to tell them the game is over . . . they are positively upset; their faces collapse. I never worry, though; they are usually the kind of people who find something else to worry about soon enough.*

"How are you, Mrs. Tannenbaum?" I asked heartily, leaving a cat who was playing a game of "Scratch My Belly."

"Terrible! Terrible! Don't ask! I just got over another coronary."

"No fooling? That's wonderful."

And then after the effort of storming in, she had to pause and slowly dip a bony finger into her pocketbook. "Excuse me," she said with a wheeze. "I've got to put another nitro under my tongue." She twisted her neck sharply, tilting her head to the side, and forced the pill down with extravagant gestures.

"Ah, that's better," she said.

The owners of the cat playing Scratch My Belly were growing impatient. The cat itself was growing impatient. And Mrs. Tannenbaum was now starting to tell me about her friend who was in traction.

I looked at the old, toothless Chihuahua, who was playing a few minor-league games with rasps and moans and obviously wanted to get into the act, and then looked on my shelf. There were some innocuous vitamin tablets there, so I gave Mrs. Tannenbaum a bottle of them and said, "One, three times a day."

"How," she asked in her incredibly raspy voice, "do I give them to him?"

"You stick them under his tongue." This is practically impossible to do with dogs. "He may give you a little trouble at first, but if you tip his head to the side like this"—I imitated her own unique twist—"and force them down like this, they'll get there. He'll love it."

And I knew that in fact the dog *would* love it, unfortunately.

Another woman came in with a cat, Charlie, who was constantly scratching his ear, a daughter in her early twenties, and a skinny little husband in his early dotage, wearing a pair of flamboyant short pants with an elastic band at the waist.

Nothing was wrong with the cat; I at once suspected he merely wanted the acknowledgment that each member of the family seemed to want. I questioned the woman while her husband and daughter stood off to the side and listened. Not only did Charlie scratch his ear, I learned, but he also cried when he had bowel movements and urinated on assorted pieces of furniture in the dining and living rooms. When the cat scratched his ear, the woman apparently took him onto her lap. Sometimes she wrapped him comfortably in a Turkish towel to check under his tongue. The cat just loved the skinless and boneless sardines she gave him for a reward afterward.

Once the history taking was complete, I had the necessary components to set up the game so they could view it from the outside. First, we playfully established the roles— I'd be the cat, the woman would be herself. Next, we needed a game board, which of course was her house; my office simulated that. What was winning? was the next question. I, playing the cat, defined winning as having the woman take me onto her lap, wrap me in a Turkish towel, and look into my mouth. Finally, we agreed on the rules. The woman agreed to do all of the above whenever I scratched my ear or cried.

By the time I'd sat on the woman's lap, simulated being wrapped in a Turkish towel, and had her play with the inside of my mouth, they were all laughing merrily. And then I brought a halt to our game. Charlie, I explained, was running her life with his ears, mouth, penis, and rectum—just as I was in the hypothetical game we had created. As long as she persisted in responding to all the cat's *signals* the way she did, the cat would, of course, continue to give her those signals. "After all," I asked, "don't you think all that feels great? I'd certainly like to come back as your cat in my next lifetime."

And suddenly it became clear to her that her well-meaning *caring* was generating all the problems. "Good heavens," she said. "I'm causing this whole mess by being so concerned!"

Whereupon the daughter became upset and said, "When I was a kid, it was the same deal. You never paid attention to me either, unless I was sick."

At which point the little old man in the outrageous short pants suddenly pulled out his wallet and showed me his press clippings. He'd been a bantamweight boxing champion in the 1920s, and he wanted to get his acknowledgment, too.

Some people are so caught up in the Sick-Pet Game that they might as well be unconscious. They are like machines going through programmed motions. Their dog twitches, they baby her. They hear her cough and instantly they dash into the bathroom to get her pills. They do the right thing and bring her in to the doctor because the doctor will tell them exactly what is wrong and, with the aid of modern science, cure it promptly. Then they can go home and wait patiently for the next game to begin. They tell me they're going to California by plane and want a tranquilizer for their dog. I say something ridiculous, merely to find out whether they're really awake. Maybe I say, "Then she'll miss the movie." They say, "Oh, then I guess we'd better not give her one."

There is so much unconsciousness out there that I sometimes think I could simplify my practice by having a Dr. Tanzer robot made. He'd have good gray hair, the mandatory stethoscope, and a look of benign, stolid wisdom on his face. He'd take people's money, use a term with -*itis* on the end, and make their dog yelp briefly. Then he'd smile, say that everything will be all right, and wave them out. They'd be happy.

But where would *my* fun come from?

Many owners are so impressed by the virtues of unconsciousness that they want some for their pet, too. A dozen times a week people want me to put a pet temporarily out of her misery with some tranquilizer. Several have begged me to do so. Unconsciousness is never a solution to anything, not for pets or people.

I have not taken tranquilizers for years and probably never will again. I do not want to be unconscious.

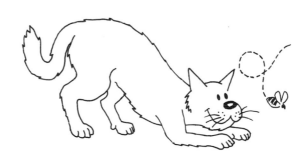

When I feel awful, I want to complete that feeling, to be done with it. Tranquilizers only produce unconsciousness and leave me feeling terrible; they prevent the feeling from going to completion and disappearing. I walk around with the feeling still in me and life becomes an endless effort to prove that I'm not awful.

"If you love your pet," I often say, "don't give her tranquilizers." Some people listen and understand, others think I don't *care*. Human beings will do anything to avoid feeling bad.

Although I prefer to use nothing, I do use something at times. When owners realize they have trained their pets to itch, scratch, twitch, lick, or urinate in the wrong place and agree to try to stop responding to these acts in their usual manner, I often lend a chemical assist by injecting the pets with a long-acting steroid. Steroids, extracts of the adrenal glands, create a state of euphoria in which the pets feel so good about themselves that they really don't need an owner or the game for about a week. In that week the owners have a chance to get out of their roles in the Sick-Pet Game and to let the pets drop their roles or acts, too.

Consciousness is what I'm after in my office—for myself, as well as for the owners and their pets.

CHAPTER 7

Who Trains Whom?

ONE OF MY DOG HILDY'S USUAL SCHEMES is biting at the skin around the base of her tail. This invariably upsets my family so much that they insist the dog has bugs. When Hildy is distraught, she begins her biting routine and I am usually forced to take her into my hospital for the day, which is probably what she wanted all the time.

Another game concerns food. I was especially anxious for Hildy to be a good eater. I like to eat, I enjoy watching Hildy eat, and bull mastiffs are *supposed* to be hearty creatures.

So when Hildy first came to the hospital with me to get rid of the bugs she didn't have, I became especially concerned when I realized I hadn't fed her that morning.

"Get me two cans of P/D," I told one of my attendants, indicating a dog food so appetizing and nutritious that I've been meaning to try it myself for some time.

Half an hour later Hildy stood pensively before a heaping plate of this marvelous stuff and said, *Yeech. Not for me.* She wouldn't touch it. She gave it barely two sniffs before she shook her head, turned up her nose, and trotted off.

I was livid. I couldn't stand her not eating. She would be big, robust, perfect—fatter than Telly Savalas's dog! She would be a bitch of stature.

Fuming, I told the attendant to go out again, this time to buy a hamburger and a potato pancake at the corner deli-catessen, known for its especially tasty food. I often eat there myself.

This time Hildy looked at the hamburger and the potato pancake, smacked her lips, and said, *Far out! The way to get the good stuff is not to eat what they put out the first time. In fact, it's also a great way to get Daddy's attention.*

Weighing the two drives—to get Daddy's attention or a quick bellyful—leads some dogs virtually to starve themselves to death. I have seen dogs who eat just enough to stay alive while their owners wear themselves out, placing before their pets perfect smorgasbords of tempting foods.

If Kitty won't eat, each night Mommy can give him a different food—shrimp, liver, smoked salmon, caviar—and play the "Gourmet Game." You can try all the different foods in the supermarket catering to this scheme—and never exhaust your pet's interest. Dogs and cats love to play this game. The more upset you get, the more you pamper your pet, the more finicky he will be.

I know.

I'm an expert at the Gourmet Game. Hildy taught it to me. Only when I can say, "That's it, Hildy. Dog food again. That's what you get and if you don't like it, *tough!*" and mean it will Hildy eat what I gave her the first time. Of course, she rather likes and usually gets two eggs—sunnyside up, if you please—crisp bacon, and two slices of buttered toast for breakfast; candy and nuts when she can steal them; and gourmet dinners. I play games, too. But I know that they *are* games, and I usually choose only the ones that are fun.

The same thing happened to thousands of owners who came to my office—but they didn't know it was a game.

"He ate well-done hamburgers for two days," a frantic cat owner tells me, "and then seemed to turn his nose up. I'm so *worried.*"

"Did you give him something else?" I ask.

"Well, we switched from ground chuck to ground round, and he ate that for a day or so, but then he turned his nose up again. I'm just beside myself. I don't know what to do."

"Well," I say, my voice very sincere, quiet, authoritative, "have you tried *boeuf* Wellington?"

The response is usually silence.

"You'll find that there's a difficult training period," I explain. "It will take a good deal of time before you learn to feed him exactly what *he* wants. And he may prefer variety. If he doesn't stay on the *boeuf* Wellington, try some *pâté de foie gras* with truffles. I know a little shop where you can get some imported from Strasbourg for only thirteen dollars a tin. Most cats like that."

The owners look at me wide-eyed.

"You don't like that?"

The owners shake their heads no, and look frightened.

"Then give him any good-quality cat food you find on the supermarket shelf—and nothing else. If he doesn't like it, tell him he can starve."

Most owners don't like that choice, either, but almost all standard brands are tasty, trustworthy, and nutritious. If you don't want to feed your pet bacon and eggs, cashews, and potato pancakes—as I let Hildy train me to do—supermarket cat food is a viable solution.

Training of all kinds is of course a central part of owning a pet . . . Such training—in a variety of forms—continues throughout a pet's entire life and is enforced by every action the owner takes that affects the animal.

Training of all kinds is of course a central part of owning a pet. There is toilet training as well as dietary training, various types of behavior conditioning, and for hunting or show dogs, very particular obedience training. Such training—in a variety of forms—continues throughout a pet's entire life and is enforced by every action the owner takes that affects the animal.

Toilet training is a fascinating—and much misunderstood—subject. The traditional way to train a dog not to urinate or defecate in the house is to rub his nose in the feces or lay out a piece of paper and praise the puppy excessively each time he uses it properly.

These methods are dead wrong.

Hundreds of cases of dogs in their middle or even late years who suddenly begin to urinate or defecate in the house again have convinced me that such training only *trains the dog to associate such actions with getting attention.* Take the case of the fox terrier who suddenly started to defecate on his owner's shoes. The man was outraged at Foxy's action, but after asking a few questions, I realized that the dog had simply put two and two together in the most natural way. If Foxy could have told me his history, it would have gone something like this:

> *This "Defecation Game" began a long time ago, Doc, when I was a little puppy. It was so nice living in this family with Mommy and Daddy. I really tried to control my bowels, but one day I had an accident and Daddy spanked me, rubbed my nose in it, and then took me and put me on an opened newspaper. Boy, were they both ever upset. I got scared, but in a little while they came over, picked me up, petted me, and Daddy said, "He's only a puppy. He didn't mean it."*
>
> *And I didn't. It was just an accident. Actually, I'd had a lot of other things on my mind, and there are certainly a lot of other things I'd like to be thinking about besides my feces. Well, after a while I could hold it long enough, and I understood that they wanted me to have my bowel movements on the paper. Every time I went on the paper, Daddy came over, hugged me, and said in his loudest voice, "Good Foxy! Terrific. You're a wonderful pup, aren't you?"*
>
> *What could I think, Doc? I'm not dumb. I can put two and two together. The way to get attention around here, real attention, is to defecate. Every time I do, they*

pet me, they give me a cookie, they treat me like roy-
alty.

Then I had a couple of really dumb accidents and
they shouted and carried on and kept watching me
every minute of the day. So I have a few more acci-
dents—frankly, Doc, these were deliberate. Well, that
did it. They began taking me to someone they called a
dog trainer, a very big man with an accent. Every time
I had an accident he shouted, "Schtop dat!" and pulled
the leash around my neck or rubbed my nose in it and
screamed at me in German. Sometimes he even hit me
with a leather strap. Boy, did I know then the power of
doo-doo! After all, I'd been totally trained that the way
to get attention is to defecate, urinate, or both. If you
do it on paper, it's good; if you do it outside, that's nice.
So I figured if I really wanted a lot of attention—like
when Daddy had been away on a business trip for three
days—I'd do it on Daddy's shoes. Can you blame me,
Doctor?

Vomiting and other such actions work the same way.

Cats, by nature, are investigative and meticulous. They
may eat a bit of broom straw. Or they lick the hair they shed
constantly because they live in a controlled environment
rather than in the wild, where they grew winter coats in the
fall and shed them every spring. They may swallow some of
the hair, which is indigestible, and this makes them vomit.
Fortunately, they've been provided with a mechanism that
enables them to vomit easily.

A family will teach a cat that if he has to vomit up a little food or some material now and then, he should do so on a piece of paper. The problem comes when they make a simple, natural act *too important*. The training is *so successful, so* filled with exclamations of "Good boy!" and with cuddling and rewards that the cat says to himself, *You know, vomiting must be desirable. It seems to work. Personally, I think it stinks, but if it turns them on, I'll try it when things get slow.*

One slow day he does try it. The cat hasn't been cuddled quite enough. He has been called "good boy" only once in five days. So he starts to vomit. His owners take it as a sure sign of terrible illness, and the game is on. It's time to play "Poor Baby." It's definitely time to visit the good veterinarian.

If you merely provide an opportunity for the pet to defecate outside or in a clean litter box and if you restrain yourself from emphasizing this simple basic function, you probably won't have a problem. Special emphasis is what causes the mischief. *You* will be creating the game from scratch. The pet will merely store the rules in his memory and revert to them when he has some sudden threat to his survival. Strive for a meld of doing nothing at all and doing what will meet the requirements of propriety and convenience—and be consistent. Harshness is often worse than neglect. Consistent actions the pet can feel certain of work.

Pets grew up for thousands of years without much help from people. Overtraining of any sort is one of the surest ways to alter their natural behavior patterns.

We tend to assume pets enjoy what we enjoy. We teach them little tricks that are fun for *us* to do or that make us proud to show off. The pet who rolls over, gets the ball, or stands on its hind legs may actually not be the smart dog. The smart dog may well be the one who does what he wants to do. *Why in hell should I want to play these dumb, ridiculous dog games?* smart Blackie must be thinking when he refuses to lie down, roll over, or beg.

> *We tend to assume pets enjoy what we enjoy . . . The smart dog may well be the one who does what he wants to do.*

"He's not very bright," the owner tells me sadly.

Nonsense, I think. That dog is brilliant.

Some dogs who do the tricks are actually adept trainers of people. When Hildy comes into the house and sits in front of me in the begging position, it may *look* as if she's doing what I taught her to do to get a cracker. I may even forget and praise myself for being such a good trainer of mischievous bull mastiffs. Actually, she's got *me* trained to give her a cracker every time she sits like that. I'm positive she's thinking, *Oh, I'll see if Daddy remembers his tricks.* So she sits, and I usually give her a cracker. I don't mind. It's a pleasant enough game—but I'd be deluding myself if I didn't know who really trained whom.

There are some startling and some subtle instances in my files of pets training their owners.

Mrs. Ringer had a fluffy little Shih Tzu who had her and her husband trained brilliantly. In fact, the dog ran their lives with a dreadful-sounding cough the way the Yorkshire terrier, Irving, in chapter 1 ran the lives of his owners. The game went on weekly, episode by episode, with the regularity and ingenuity of a soap opera.

The root of the problem lay, I thought, in the fact that Mrs. Ringer's last dog had died of congestive heart disease. She had yet to get over the loss of the other dog, so she kept experiencing her present dog through the previous dog's death.

The cough, of course, sounded serious; accompanied by a studied wheeze, it might even have been taken for congestive heart disease. This symptom was no coincidence. Mrs. Ringer used to get furious with me when I laughed at the situation; her dog *had* to be dying from that "terrible cough." He'd been dying from it for the previous ten weeks of their soap opera.

"It started," she told me, "after I started taking him to be trained." This was training to heel, accomplished with a leash that was pulled up short whenever he didn't heel. "Oh, it's dreadfully upsetting, Doctor," she said. "Can't you do something? Last night he woke Melvin and me at two in the morning. We had to get out of bed and look down his throat. It sounded exactly as if there was something stuck there. I was so terrified that he was going to choke that we stayed up most of the night."

"You took the dog to a trainer who taught him—and you—the use of a leash," I told her. "But the training also taught your dog some other tricks. The first time you pulled that leash up short, he probably choked a little and coughed; it hurt. And you probably bent over and asked if he was all right. After that, whenever he coughed you probably stopped pulling on the leash. Right?"

"Yes, that's so."

"The dog now thinks, *I hate this ridiculous game. Walking around the block, the same block, endlessly, and getting nearly choked every few steps.* So he coughs and trains you to stop pulling on the leash. He's trained you to know that he prefers to be walked gently, not pulled, and he's done it all by coughing. Not only that, but you're now upset because you're sure you've hurt him. *Ah-ha*, thinks the dog. *I'll play this to the hilt. Whenever I want Mommy or Daddy to pick me up and worry about me and comfort me, I'll cough. It's an exciting new game. I love it.*"

One dog, I told Mrs. Ringer, had even trained its owner to *count* by coughing. She could tell me that the dog had coughed precisely *sixty-three* times the night before. When the dog coughed *Chuaugh,* the owner said, "One!"

Chuaugh!

"Two!"

Chuaugh!

"Three!"

Only the owner didn't get a biscuit for learning, just aggravation and worry.

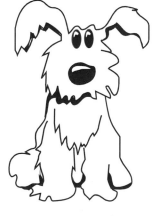

Mrs. Ringer finally stopped worrying about the cough, which was purely an act, and miraculously, it disappeared. Dozens of other owners, however, spend the better part of their lives doing tricks their pets have taught them.

One dog says to a visiting dog friend, *Hey, watch this great new trick I taught Mommy. I'm going to give her a signal, and she's going to go immediately to that cabinet in the bathroom, open it up, take out one of those white pills from the little bottle, come over and hold me around the neck, and shove this thing down. It's terrific. Now watch.*

And he says *Arrrh-arr, arrgh-arr* in a very special way and wrenches his neck back a little, and Mommy throws up her hands and goes directly to the bathroom as if she were a toy train chugging on tracks.

When he's got the pill down, the dog looks over proudly at his friend and says, *See? Isn't she well trained? It only took a couple of weeks to teach her that.*

Well, the friend says—he's a plump Airedale with a savvy look in his eye—*my Mommy is a swell toy, too. I know exactly what buttons to push. I grunt a lot while I am having a bowel movement. Actually, I sort of enjoy enemas right now.*

That is another story.

If you must be your pet's best toy, I tell some owners, at least be aware of what you're doing. Choose to play when you want to play. Don't be a robot.

Having read this far, you might want to be sure of where you stand with your own pets. To find out, answer the following questions as honestly as possible—and come up with your own conclusions.

- Has your dog trained you to take him out late at night?

- What are three good tricks you've learned?

- Have you expanded your culinary skills since your dog showed you how he likes his food?

- Has your dog made you a selective shopper?

- Has your cat trained you to read cat-food labels?

- Has your dog trained you to get up at 6:00 in the morning to prevent him from defecating on the rug, because he doesn't particularly want to wait until 7:30 to play with you?

- Have you learned how to play "Chase the Pet" when it's pill-taking time?

These are all good games. But you ought to choose whether you want to play them or not, don't you think?

CHAPTER 8

Over to the Left and Down a Little

WHEN THE WOMAN PUT TRIXIE, a gorgeous gray tabby cat, on the examining table, the animal looked at me a moment and said, *Wait until you see this!*

She was an elegant cat, with measured, delicate movements, and she took a choice position on the table, arched her back, and raised her tail straight up. The backs of her thighs were almost entirely hairless. Trixie displayed the area boldly and asked, *Well, what do you think of* that?

I knew what the owner thought of it. The owner liked to exhibit this cat every year in a local cat-fancier's show. There were awards for the handsomest cat, but there were none for the cat with the barest rump. The owner was upset and frightened. Why had her Trixie caught this terrible skin disease two weeks before the show?

Trixie had what is usually called linear granuloma, a chronic inflammatory lesion on a pet's upper thighs. Skin lesions and various forms of skin disease like this one are common in pets.

The problem had started three weeks earlier, shortly after the woman had adopted a little yellow kitten from the pound. "Trixie must have caught it from her," the woman said. "Don't you think so?"

Having explored thousands of similar cases, it was immediately clear to me what had happened. "It didn't start three weeks ago" I told the woman. "This problem started *four years ago* when Trixie was born."

The woman couldn't understand.

I explained to her that being born is a terrifying experience for any animal. At first she's floating in a delicious balloon, with all her needs satisfied. Then suddenly this comfortable time is over, and the kitten or puppy—or any other newborn, for that matter—must begin to fend for herself. The newcomer is thrust into a narrow tunnel that nearly crushes her. There are strange lights, noises, frightening sensations, and pain. The newcomer is terrified she won't survive. But she does survive—and her survival is accompanied by some

> *I explained to her that being born is a terrifying experience for any animal . . . The newcomer is terrified she won't survive. But she does . . .*

important events. The first thing that happens after the
shock and the threat of death is that the mother *licks* the kitten or puppy, especially around its genitalia. While the young
animal nurses—itself a pleasurable experience instinctively
associated with survival—the mother cleans away the excrement, removing any scents or odors that might attract preda-
tors. This licking stimulates the kitten or puppy to have its
first bowel movement and to urinate. These instinctive
actions by the mother permanently link the survival experience with the feeling of an animal's tongue licking it. This
experience, like all experiences, is stored in the animal's
mind (its "computer").

The woman thought this idea was a little far-fetched.
Why, she wanted to know, did Trixie start licking the
inflamed areas right after the new kitten arrived home from
the pound? "Trixie must have *caught* something from that
kitten!"

"The new kitten was the trigger," I explained. "Trixie
needed you. She'd spent four marvelous years with you. She
felt safe. You were her whole world. Then suddenly you were
all excited about this adorable little thing you'd gotten from
the pound. Trixie feared for her survival and automatically
recalled her earliest "tapes" on survival, starting with her
birth experience. She programmed her computer to deal with
the perceived threat to and her desire for survival, and the
result was a memory of a cat's tongue licking her all over,
especially around her rump. So she chose the first available
tongue, which happened to be her own, and began to lick.

"Cats' tongues are coarse as sandpaper, and it wasn't long
before Trixie's licked derriere was hairless and irritated. The

more attention you paid to the kitten's cute antics the more Trixie licked. Then she jumped up onto a table one day, lifted her tail—as she did here in the office—and you saw it, that terrible skin disease. You were alarmed and worried. You examined the area carefully and looked at it often. The more you looked, the more old Trixie licked. She was, indeed, surviving with all this regained attention."

Let me hold off suggesting what to do—or more accurately, what *not* to do—in such cases until later chapters. For the moment let me merely point out the causes of most licking problems and skin disease: (1) recollection of the birth experience, and (2) attention from the owner, the reward that keeps the problem going. Most of the "skin disease" I have seen follows this simple pattern. Usually the only variations are the events that trigger the onset of licking and the nature of the owner's response.

For instance, I often wondered why skin lesions were such a large problem in the summertime, when I would see hundreds of cases a week. The common assumption is that summer dermatitis, or "hot spots," is caused by allergies. But such lesions do not exactly correspond to the so-called allergy season. However, the season does, I suspect, duplicate the conditions of temperature and humidity that the wet, newborn animal felt just after it completed its earliest survival experience. Reminded of how great the world seemed then, the animal attempts to duplicate those pleasurable feelings and *automatically* begins to lick. The owner *automatically* begins to look and to touch. And the pet thinks, *Ah! That feels great. I selected the right tape from my memory bank. Scratch me over to the left and down a little.*

The game is on.

Why are skin lesions so common?

Maybe it's because being born is so common.

CHAPTER 9

Defecating to Survive

FULLY 50 PERCENT OF THE CASES I have treated revolve around the anal orifice. A good number are caused by itching and scratching and licking; many are directly connected to excrement. For pets, excrement is often a prime weapon in the arsenal of survival. In other words, many pets defecate to survive.

When the cat urinates on Harvey's newly pressed suit, he may be doing so because he loves Harvey—who, I learned, had come home that night so his wife could go off to class for the first time. Harvey's curses and even the beating he delivered (which he atoned for by special warmth toward the cat) only convinced the animal that he had chosen the right way to get attention.

Cats and dogs do not think feces are "bad." We do. Here are a few examples of this human aversion. There are "antidefecation leagues" in dozens of cities (people who, it often seems to me, are delighted to have the Defecation Game to get upset about). From time to time medical authorities claim that children will go blind from exposing their optic nerves to the fumes from pet excrement. For a while researchers thought that if pregnant women got within twenty-five yards of a kitty litter pan, she'd get toxoplasmosis and give birth to an imbecile. Finally, the development of Superdooper Pooper-Scoopers suggests that without too much difficulty, a vast industry could quickly grow up around dog feces.

Pet defecation may not be a threat to the optic nerves, but it does cause traumatic reactions. One very sad young woman came in with a brown-and-white terrier, whom she wanted to have destroyed. The dog was less than a year old. "I can't stand him any more," she said.

"You want me to *kill* this dog?" I asked, terribly upset at the prospect. I knew I wouldn't do what she wanted, but if she was committed to the act, someone else might.

"I love the dog," she said tearfully, "but he's urinating all over the house."

She was a schoolteacher, and the problem had started the day after she started school in September. She'd also bought a new rug from Bloomingdale's with a huge rose in the middle, and it was that rug, which she'd wanted to buy for years, that had been ruined.

Clearly, from the moment that rug had arrived, it meant trouble for Georgie. He'd been locked in the kitchen while the men unrolled it. Sophie from next door, who usually brought him soup bones, came over to look at that rug instead. Worst of all, Mommy suddenly wasn't home all day.

What's going on here? the dog must have thought. *I don't think I like this scene.*

An animal's mental computer is wired for survival in different ways. For some animals, fear for survival and wanting to survive brings up licking on any part of the body. For others, it brings up the urination that accompanied the mother's licking of the newborn's genitals at its birth. Georgie's computer told him to urinate and he promptly began to do so on Mommy's new rug from Bloomingdale's.

At three o'clock, when the owner returned from school, she found the yellow stains on her white rug right next to the rose. She chased the dog, shouted, whacked him. The dog then decided to try the corner of the sofa. This place worked even better! Mommy was nearly hysterical now.

The dog clearly had lots of proof that urinating was the way to get attention—and attention for pets equals survival. If this behavior continued, it would be a difficult pattern to break. Even human beings are reluctant to give up a survival pattern that works. Feeling fear and anger and acting in some asocial way may be viewed as negative but at least one is feeling and being something. *Nothing* is unfamiliar; it's like blank space. Better to feel something negative than to feel nothing.

> *The dog clearly had lots of proof that urinating was the way to get attention—and attention for pets equals survival. If this behavior continued, it would be a difficult pattern to break.*

The carpet was ruined, so I recommended that the woman allow the dog to continue urinating on it. But every time he urinated, she was to silently pick him up without a fuss and put him in the bathroom by himself for an hour.

She might give him some encouragement for going in the right place but nothing demonstrative. The dog was still quite young and might break the pattern quickly if he saw that the reaction was indifference and the effect, isolation, was unpleasant.

Fortunately he did break his behavior pattern. But if the dog had persisted, he would have been *right* in his choice of a game that worked, but he would have been dead.

Ironically, the enthusiasm that led to his death would have been the result of his efforts to survive.

There was a wealthy tycoon who owned an Airedale. Like the man's wife, the Airedale was fairly high-strung. All of them were extremely handsome. The man was a dynamo; he employed nearly a hundred people and ran his world with an iron fist.

His fairly high-strung wife brought the fairly high-strung Airedale to my office one day some time ago, complaining about his loose bowel movements. I examined the dog and could find no organic problems. So I began my standard investigation.

I discovered that nine days earlier the woman had been painting the living room. She had shouted at the dog, "Get out of here! You're going to get full of paint!" Soon afterward the dog's diarrhea started—in the middle of the carpet.

Now that I knew the history of the problem, I was able to explain it. I told the woman quietly that the dog loved her, needed her for survival, and when he grew upset, his intestines reacted. He wanted attention and he got it with his diarrhea.

The woman laughed lightly and said she couldn't possibly believe that; the problem had to be organic.

I told her my examination of the dog proved otherwise.

But how, she wanted to know—and it was surely a good question—could he possibly have learned *how* to have diarrhea and that having it was a way to get attention?

Now that I knew the history of the problem, I was able to explain it. I told the woman quietly that the dog loved her, needed her for survival, and when he grew upset, his intestines reacted. He wanted attention and he got it with his diarrhea.

I took a stab at an answer. "When he was a puppy, he had a problem with diarrhea, didn't he?"

"Yes."

"Did you look at his bowel movements?"

"Yes. The vet we were seeing then told us we had to watch and be able to describe the stool."

"Did you check every bowel movement?" I asked.

"Most of them. Ugh. Jerry checked some."

"I suspect," I said, "that he decided the way to Mommy's and Daddy's hearts is through his excrement. Every time he defecated, somebody looked. It worked once, when he was a puppy, so now when he's suddenly afraid, he tries it again. He has a loose bowel movement and—guess what?—you prove he's right. You put down the paint brush and come over, and he says, *Absolutely marvelous. It works.*"

"Look," she said, "I am not about to go home and tell my husband *that*. He'll throw me out."

"Fine," I said. "Then we'll treat it like a *real* disease." And I gave the dog a standard injection and the woman some corrective medication to give him twice daily, and in a few days she was through with her painting and the dog was fine.

It was a wonderful cure.

But a few weeks later, the Airedale was back, this time with the tycoon. The dog was limping. This character was more versatile than Robert DeNiro; he had a dozen roles. Now the dog was playing a wounded nobleman returning to Moscow from the Russo-Japanese war.

There was nothing at all wrong with his leg. But I learned that when he was a puppy, he'd been stepped on. Act 1, the diarrhea, had stopped working; so he'd gone on to act 2, being lame.

The tycoon roared with laughter when I proposed this theory. "Listen," he said, "my wife told me what you said. I think you're nuts."

"Great," I said. "But tell me more about his anal history."

I soon learned that he'd sent the dog several times to a highly authoritarian trainer. The owner was a man who really ran his world. He had a superb specimen of an Airedale, and this defecating, I could see, was an affront to his pride. He'd never liked it. He was glad it was over now. He could live with the limp, especially since I'd now assured him it was not serious.

Although the dog had decided after a while that it was simpler to defecate outside than to be sent back to the brutal trainer, he was a high-strung animal and apparently reverted to old attention-getting devices whenever he was upset. Throughout his life, every time he had a bowel movement in

the right place, he was praised. Every time he had an accident, he was shouted at and his nose was shoved into the
mess. This "training" produced a dog whose attention was
tightly focused on his own anus.

The fact that the dog had diarrhea, presumably a *real* disease, may seem puzzling. Solid stools often *become* loose as
the game-playing becomes more important to the animal,
more desperate. Loose stool looks like a real disease. As the
animal learns that the way to get attention is to defecate, it
makes an automatic assumption that more is better; so it
expels another, then another, stool.

The mechanical arrangement of the intestinal tract is
such that, as a bowel movement comes down into the lower
part of the bowel, water is reabsorbed from it and it is solidi-
fied. But if the animal keeps pushing the stool out before it
gets a chance to spend any time in the rectum, the water is
not reabsorbed and the stool comes out loose. It comes out
too early, full of mucous, and looks patently abnormal. *Hysterical* disease has thus been contrived to mimic real organic
disease perfectly. To succeed in dominating the owner, the
dog must be a convincing con artist.

I was not at all surprised to hear that the Airedale had
a recurrence of diarrhea a few weeks later and that the
owner had taken him to a large animal medical center,
where dozens of interns and doctors walked around offi-
ciously with badges and clipboards. He had paid over
$1,500 for an extensive battery of "conclusive tests." The
owner was the kind of man who trafficked daily in hard,
realistic facts. He was willing to pay a great deal to get
them.

However, the medical center couldn't give him the facts he wanted. The tests uncovered nothing. The problem persisted.

When the man came back to me, I told him, "I had a woman in here once who told me her puppy had defecated seventeen times in the previous two days. She had a chart, with the time and place written down for each instance. You're not that bad, but you've trained this dog to think that the way to your heart is through his anus."

This time he took a chance; he believed me. But when I proposed (omitting the usual role-playing game with him)

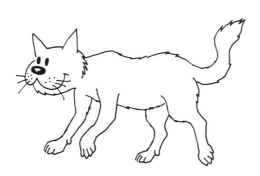

that he and his wife were directly causing the diarrhea, he scoffed. "I run a small empire—and you're telling me this dog is running my life with his asshole, that *I'm* causing it?"

"That's it."

He thought for a moment. "Well, maybe so," he said in a subdued voice.

"When it becomes perfectly all right for your dog to defecate," I told him, "he'll probably stop. I don't know whether you're willing to live with the problem. Some people wouldn't. They'd get rid of the dog and try again. If you rub his nose in it, you'll only be saying, 'See? This is why I'm paying attention to you.' You've got to leave it and him alone. You shouldn't even clean it up in front of him. Try whistling when he defecates. If possible, do even less. The dog can *smell* when you're upset—and being upset with him is a form of attention."

I think the man understood. He ran his world well because he had learned to listen. And he told me that he practiced my lessons scrupulously well. In several weeks the problem vanished, with the help of steroids (which provided some temporary euphoria for the little terrorist).

On his way out of my office that day he met a woman coming in with a dog who happened to limp and have diarrhea. "Hold on a minute," he said to her. "Tell me that again." She did, and since she looked like a good sport, he took over the examination and advised, "You don't need Tanzer. I'll tell you what the problem is." And he did so with enthusiasm. "That's the whole story," he said, "and the key point is that you're causing it all. He's going to tell you exactly the same thing, and it's going to cost you fifty bucks." He paused. "But it may be the cheapest fifty you'll ever spend."

CHAPTER 10

Fat Dog, Thin Dog

THE BEAGLE COULD HARDLY GET THROUGH the door. She looked like a piggy bank. I'd never seen a dog so overweight.

A young man had called me about the case that morning, saying, "You have to do me a favor and help me get my parents to stop overfeeding that dog. Cakes from Elfenbaum's. Knishes. Table scraps. *Whole* meals from the table! The animal is ridiculous."

She certainly was. As soon as I saw her—and the plump little couple who waddled into my office after her—I looked up suddenly and announced in my most stentorian tones, "This dog has approximately three months to live if you don't stop overfeeding her!"

That ought to scare them, I thought to myself.

The woman looked at me and without a moment's delay, without changing her sweet-little-old-lady expression one iota, said, "If she's only got three months to live, at least during her last three months she should be happy and eat well."

People especially conscious of fatness or thinness—for any of a thousand reasons—may find that their pets will resort to one or the other extreme because it elicits their owners' keenest attention.

The beagle was not a unique case. I once read the riot act to another couple with an obese Chihuahua crossbreed. At first they swore that they hadn't been overfeeding the little blimp. They insisted the trouble must be the result of glands or of the dog's having been spayed.

It is amazing to me how readily people will accept false causes because they *sound* logical or scientific.

But the true causes for the Chihuahua's weight problem came out within a few moments. Under repeated questioning, little by little, the couple admitted that they fed the dog half a slice of bread now and then and a snack in the evening. The Chihuahua should have weighed six pounds; she weighed thirty. Half a slice of bread constituted half the dog's daily caloric needs.

I looked at the couple. They were a trim enough, athletic pair. They seemed to have no dietary problems.

I looked at the dog. Every breath was a struggle. The effort the plump little thing had to go through just to stay alive!

"Well, you see how fat she is," I said. "Neither glands nor spaying caused this." I pointed a finger at them both. "You—"

"Oh, no," the woman interrupted. "It's not really us. It's Grandpa!"

"Grandpa?" I asked. Here was a new player in the drama.

"He's so hooked on the dog," the man said, "that when we say the dog needs exercise, Grandpa *drives* her to the park so she won't have to walk."

I met Grandpa some weeks later. He weighed over two hundred pounds and huffed and puffed like an old steam locomotive each time he took a step.

Dr. William Kay, chief of staff of the Animal Medical Center in New York City, was recently quoted in the *New York Times*: "I've observed that often overweight pets are owned by overweight people." The "coincidence," he explained, is lack of dietary control for both the pet and owner.

Obviously, both gain weight because they eat too much; that's usually the way one gains weight. But the *cause* lies deeper. The "coincidence," if you believe even one-tenth of what I've written here, is scarcely a coincidence.

Fat people *create* fat pets. They may do so to make it all right to be fat or in order to vent their hostility toward obesity on this nearby creature. Fat people also create *thin* dogs to experience thinness, at least in some member of the family.

Fat and thin dogs, dogs with dietary abnormalities, are often working a con game uniquely keyed to their owners' sensitivities. People especially conscious of fatness or thinness—for any of a thousand reasons—may find that their pets will resort to one or the other extreme because it elicits their owners' keenest attention. In effect, the owners are creating the abnormalities. I cannot always decipher the reasons, but I can usually spot a game that's being played. It's not always easy, though.

In one case, Duke, a bull mastiff, had not eaten any food in three weeks. He had lost a full fifty pounds. Nothing his owners could do, not all their desperate pleas and force-feedings, could alter the dog's will not to eat.

The couple were almost ready to give the dog away. They couldn't bear to see him starving. I knew the man had recently quit his job. I also knew that they were thoughtful people who loved this animal. They were beside themselves. They'd even taken to forcing open his mouth and squirting in milk and other liquid food.

The problem, I learned, began while they were caring for the dog after a minor operation. The dog had the saddest look on his face I've ever seen on an animal. The couple were heartbroken by that look. Even in my office they couldn't help saying, "Poor Baby" to the dog every few minutes. (It's intensely interesting to me that *nice* people usually have the greatest number of problems with their pets. Mean people don't care. They neglect their pets when they're ill and the animals then rapidly recover.)

The problem with this bull mastiff *might* be physical, I thought, and I gave him, as usual, a thorough physical examination before coming to any conclusions.

The results were negative. I could find nothing at all wrong with the dog.

I suggested to the couple that the dog *might* be getting more nurturing by *not* eating than he was by eating. The attention he got might be more important to him than food. In such terms, he was surely "winning" his particular—and certainly peculiar—game. By the time they left that day, they had agreed to try my prescription of "nothing"; they would not try to feed the dog and would not pay it any particular attention when it did not eat.

A few days later the man called up and said, "Dr. Tanzer, there's really something terribly wrong with this dog. We've been doing what you said, but the situation just isn't improving. The dog won't eat. The whole family's desperately worried. Maybe we should give the dog away."

I had them bring the dog in again, examined it, found noth-

I suggested to the couple that the dog might be getting more nurturing by not eating than he was by eating. The attention he got might be more important to him than food. In such terms, he was surely "winning" his particular— and certainly peculiar— game.

ing, and then decided I'd better do a really thorough workup. I hated to take their money. I felt sure the problem was not organic, but I was beginning to wonder whether I hadn't missed something. I could be wrong. I had to be sure. So I gave the dog chest, skull, and abdominal x-rays. I ordered a red blood count, a white-cell count, a differential count, and hemoglobin and hematocrit tests, as well as kidney-function and liver-function tests.

When I got the results, I could see that the kidney-function test results were slightly off. But when I double-checked this with still another test, I realized that this problem was insignificant. The dog was really perfectly normal. The test results reaffirmed my initial clinical impression.

"We hate to give him up," the woman said, "but there's no way we can live with this much longer. We'd love to keep him, but he makes us anxious, you know. And all these visits and tests are . . . well . . . expensive."

I suspected but could not say that they really *did* want to get rid of the dog. People reach such moments; financial and emotional matters combine with the special pressures in a given household and the pet becomes the scapegoat. At such times, owners may even create special problems in their animals that will justify giving the pet up or having it put to sleep.

"There's nothing wrong with this dog, I assure you," I told them. "This is a healthy dog, a good dog. But for some reason he's playing a bad game. You've got to make it all right for this dog to die. If he's intent on starving himself to death, he'll do so whether you *care* or not. I think he's giving you the business. I think if you good people will stop *caring* so much, he'll stop this act. But you should be prepared. He may persist. And if he does, he'll prove that he's right, and he'll die."

Though they promised to try, I was not at all sure when they left the office that I wouldn't hear from them again soon. The case was complex, the owners did not seem fully convinced about my ideas, and they seemed to be unclear not only about the "cure" but about whether they wanted to keep the dog.

A few days later I recognized the man's anxious voice on the phone again. "He's not any better."

"Are you sure you're doing what I said?"

"Well, Gertie gives him some chicken soup with a bulb syringe four or five times a day and . . . "

"Stop!"

"Wha-at?"

"You're not doing *nothing*! Shoving soup into a dog's mouth with a bulb syringe is not doing *nothing*. Look, why don't you bring the dog in and leave him with me for a few days? There may be something I can do, either here or at my home if I have him to myself. It's an interesting case. There won't be any charge."

They were willing to do this and even told me when they appeared with the dog that they were delighted to leave their delinquent at the "Tanzer Camp for Disturbed Dogs." I welcomed the challenge. I hoped to cure the dog by using my threats and the benign influence of the notorious glutton Hildy.

I had a busy caseload the morning they brought the woefully shrunken bull mastiff into my office. At first I merely left him some food. He wouldn't touch it. Later I tried to trick him by tossing a few bits of toast into the air. Instinctively he grabbed them, but he only chewed them, then spit them out. I thought I caught his eyes watching me. If he was acting, he could have won an Oscar. I was puzzled. It *had* to be an act. I doubted by now that I could discover *why* this game was being played, but I had to know *if* the dog was playing a game.

An hour later, in anger—since I'm quite human and often forget my own best advice about doing nothing—I tried to stuff some food down his throat. He would have none of it. Stuffing never works.

That afternoon, when I had a free half-hour, I decided on a showdown. I told one of my attendants to go out and buy two meatloaf sandwiches. When he returned, I put them down in front of the dog, established eye contact, glared at him, and said, "Look, I think you're a wretched fake. But if you *really* want to die, that's exactly what I'm going to help

you do. I'm going to take you home, take you into my back-
yard, and dig a big, beautiful hole. It will be to bury you in,
mister. If that's what you want, that's what you'll get. You're
causing too much trouble. Get that? Now *eat*! Eat this food
or you're going to end up in that hole."

The dog didn't budge.

"Well, maybe you want to save face and eat when I'm not
around," I said, walking just outside the door.

A little later, when I peeked in, the dog was wolfing
down both meatloaf sandwiches. He looked up briefly at me,
met my eyes, then finished munching.

And that evening, after I'd decided to leave the dog in
the hospital another day before taking him home, I caught
him sneaking into the bathroom, where a moment later, he
was slurping madly from the toilet bowl.

"What a fraud!" I thought. "What a charlatan."

But I was wrong. The dog couldn't help himself.

The story, unfortunately, has a sad but revealing ending.

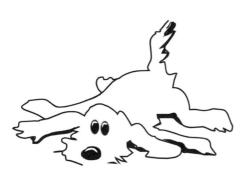

In the ensuing months, I
learned that the man had
created this problem to play
out a larger drama in his
life. He had switched pro-
fessions from a stable job to
a chancy career in the arts
and wanted to be free from
the responsibilities of his family.

The dog developed a series of complicated maladies, cul-
minating in severe paralysis of his left side for which I could
find no organic cause. Despite my pleas, the man now

insisted that I put his dog to sleep. I offered to treat the animal as long as necessary; he could pay me in a year, whenever he could. I even offered to keep the dog in my hospital for a time at no charge.

He refused my offers. He wanted the dog killed. I stalled, but finally did what he wanted.

On the day he came in to pick up the body, my secretary tried to console him. She was sorry, she said, Duke had been a wonderful dog. The man needed none of her condolences. He was absolutely delighted! He had symbolically encapsulated all of his unwanted responsibilities in the pet and then destroyed them.

What a pity that such a fine dog had to be sacrificed to this man's blind drama!

CHAPTER 11

Pain

MANY OWNERS WILL GO TO ABSURD LENGTHS to avoid seeing their pets in pain or even discomfort. This is a common phenomenon in my office, a dangerous syndrome, and it no doubt indicates that the owners have simply not recognized that pain is an inevitable part of life and that avoiding it will only cause the drama of fearing pain to persist. Such owners demand tranquilizers and general anesthesia for their pets; they turn their heads away when I give injections, and they plead with me not to butcher poor Wowser.

If such owners can be given the experience of pain, if they can be allowed to see that they can bear it and survive, their fear may even disappear.

Not long ago I had a trembling woman in my office with a young female poodle who was also trembling visibly. The woman lived in terror of physicians, and so did her dog, apparently. She had ostensibly brought the dog, Tammy, to get booster injections, but I

felt she was really creating a drama—a good one, actually—
so she could stop playing this game she'd learned when she
was eight years old and got hurt in a doctor's office. She was
ready to face the pain but didn't
know whether she could. She
wanted to experience it, survive,
and be done with this particular
drama. She wanted doctors'
offices to be less awesome places
for her. That's how I perceived
her situation.

*Many owners will go to
absurd lengths to avoid
seeing their pets in pain or
even discomfort. This is a
common phenomenon . . .
and it no doubt indicates
that the owners have sim-
ply not recognized that
pain is an inevitable part
of life and that avoiding it
will only cause the drama
of fearing pain to persist.*

I set out to let her know that
I understood and wanted her to
experience the event completely.
She watched me establish eye
contact with her dog and calm
her, and this calmed the woman. "Now I want you to watch
me give the dog these booster injections," I said firmly.

"I couldn't bear it!" she said, her hands coming up to her
face.

I told her she could. I was sure of it. I did not resist her
fear; I did not tell her she was wrong to be afraid. But I gave
her the opportunity—and she took it.

I did not insert the first syringe until she came several
steps closer and promised not to turn her eyes away. The
injection took a few seconds. She watched with only a slight
flinch. The next shot caused no flinch at all.

When she left, something in her voice as she thanked
me—audible strength and confidence—made me feel I'd
served her well.

Consider the following extreme—but far from unusual—
case: A man and a woman, new clients, brought in their
miniature schnauzer, who had a broken toenail. The nail was
broken beneath the quick. It was hanging partially attached,
and it must have been somewhat painful to the little animal.
Clearly, it had to be removed, and the quickest, simplest
method was to take a pair of surgical pliers and give a quick
yank. This procedure would cause no more pain than the
original trauma that broke the nail.

I looked up from the table at the owners. The wife was a
fluttery women in frilly clothes, about fifty years old; there
was pain in her face—and fear. Her husband, who stood to
one side, had an obvious neurological problem that distorted
his face. He had, no doubt, lived for some time with great
pain. He said nothing, but she kept chattering away nervously. "He's in terrible pain with his nail. You can see that,
can't you, Doctor? You won't hurt him, will you? I don't want
you to hurt him. I don't want him to have any pain. We love
him so. I don't know how he hurt his poor little nail. We
noticed it this morning and came right over. He's in very, very
terrible pain, isn't he, Doctor?"

"It hurts him a little," I said. "I'll have to remove the
nail." I felt a sudden urge to put a tongue depressor into her
mouth, so she couldn't talk during the rest of the examination.

"Don't hurt him!"

"Well, it *is* going to hurt a little."

"Oh, can't you give him an anesthetic? I don't want him
to have any pain whatsoever. I couldn't bear that." Her hands

came up to her face. The pitch of her voice grew higher. "Can't you do *something*, Doctor?"

Was all this fuss really about a broken toenail? I knew it wasn't. I'd seen scores of owners act in similar, if slightly less hysterical, ways. Several owners just that morning had literally begged me to give their pets tranquilizers. I had refused.

Clearly, though, my real problem was not to deal with the schnauzer's pain, so much as with this woman's almost fanatical aversion to pain. I could best serve this woman— and her pet—by strengthening her ability to confront pain. If she didn't complete this drama in her life, she was sure to create a lot of bad games in her miniature schnauzer. The dog would simply have to play the Sick-Dog Game, when all that juicy concern and worry were the inevitable reward.

"We can do one of two things," I said, knowing I would only do one of them. "If you insist upon anesthesia, we can take this animal into the hospital and put him under general anesthesia. This will involve his staying for at least twenty-four hours. He'll need some preoperative work-up so we can see if he can tolerate the anesthetic, and I would be remiss not to warn you that there is definitely some risk to his life with general anesthesia."

Some veterinarians, at the first sign of discomfort in an owner, would not merely suggest, but actually recommend, this alternative. "Certainly I can remove the nail painlessly," I said, "with the help of general anesthesia."

I looked at them both. They were not rich people.

"And all this," I said, "will cost approximately five to ten times what it would cost to handle the situation another way."

The woman nodded.

I looked at her husband. He had not said a word. He stood, shaking slightly, his face partially distorted. Whatever violent neurological disturbance he'd had—perhaps a stroke—had left him crippled and perhaps unable to speak properly.

"Or," I continued, "you can grit your teeth, and I can restrain the dog for a moment or two, grab the nail with pliers . . . "

"*Nooooo!*" The woman's voice was a low wail, sad and terrified.

" . . . yank the nail, and it's all over. Then you can take him home. And this will cost twenty dollars. Which shall I do?"

Without hesitation she said, "I just can't do it to the poor little thing." Her voice was low and soft, trembling slightly but perfectly resolved. "No, I do not want him hurt in any way. I'll leave him here, Doctor, and you have him put under

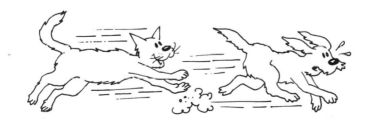

anesthesia while you do what has to be done. That won't hurt a bit, will it? I've been under general anesthesia three times, and I felt nothing. Nothing at all. It was just like being asleep."

I was astounded at her decision.

Her husband was even more deeply affected. He, who obviously was no stranger to far more severe pain than we were dealing with here, grew livid. With jerky, tense motions he began to move toward her. I could scarcely understand the garbled words that came from his contorted lips, but it looked as if he might attack his wife physically—if he didn't collapse first.

I had scarcely expected this intense reaction on his part. I felt a bolt of fear myself and shouted, "Stop! Hold it this instant!"

The man backed away, grasping the edge of a cabinet.

"Look," I said, my voice authoritative now. I looked directly at the stricken man. "There is no way I'm going to do what she wants me to do. Relax. *Please*."

Then I looked at the woman. She began to cry. I said, "I am not going to jeopardize this animal's life. I will not under any circumstances give it general anesthesia in the service of stopping that little *yeeep* of pain."

I looked at the man. He was calmer now. I asked the woman to consider how inappropriate her decision was, how extreme were the lengths to which she would go to avoid confronting pain.

She looked at me and said with a touch of defiance, with a sure sense that she not only had fears but she certainly wasn't going to be talked out of them. "Well, that's the way I am. I'm sorry. I just can't stand pain. I will not allow you to hurt my dog."

I was becoming angry. "You're going to stand right here," I said, pointing to the exact spot and speaking with exaggerated control. "Right here. Right now. And you're going to watch every gesture I make. I am going to pull this dog's toenail off, and you're going to see me do it."

Her hands went to her face. She said, "I can't."

"Nonsense!" When her hands came away from her face, I took the pliers and gave a quick yank. The dog gave a little *yeeep*—and it was all over.

"That's it," I said, feeling satisfied that I had done the best thing for both the dog and the owners.

She stood silently, pain draining visibly from her face. When I told her that she probably created problems for herself that badly complicated her life, she nodded. When I asked her if the event had been too traumatic for her, she shook her head no. I told her to think of what she could have done because of her flight from pain. "You might have gotten this animal killed," I told her, "trying to prevent his having a little pain."

Her face was relaxed now. She had seen the drama through. I had the distinct impression that she would handle pain differently now, whenever it touched her life.

CHAPTER 12

Postoperative Noncare

THE HUGE COLLIE, weighing a good 120 pounds, had eaten a bar of Dial soap. He was pouring blood out rectally and vomiting; he was terribly dehydrated. It was gastroenteritis. The collie was dying; there was no doubt about it. The family had waited for four days to bring him in, and they were all profoundly guilt stricken and hysterical.

Was there *any* chance at all? "Oh, if *only* you can save Weepy ... Cost is no object. Anything. Just save him."

This was many years ago. I had recently graduated from Cornell, and I felt that dogs who managed to die on me had fantastic nerve. I wouldn't let them die. I already had a reputation for diagnosing and curing hard cases, and I loved the chance to do highly sophisticated surgery, to work all night with seemingly terminal dogs and ultimately save them.

This was an impossible case.

Great, I thought. I could play Supervet.

I remember comforting the family, advising them that they should expect the worst, taking the collie into the hospital and rolling up my sleeves. I attacked the case with intravenous drips, immediately. I medicated and hydrated, administered subcutaneous feeding, and treated the dog constantly for five days. I wasn't going to be beaten by a bar of Dial soap.

Several times the family came in, stood near the cage watching Weepy, and cried their eyes out. He was a scraggly, ugly, foul-smelling dog, but they loved him. "Doctor," they asked, watching the poor dog lying listlessly on the floor of the cage, "are you sure you've done *everything?*"

I was sure. But in spite of all my efforts the dog lay there dying.

"Save our poor baby!" they pleaded, and I tried. I struggled and struggled, but this dog's case seemed to be too much for me. *I'm going to die,* he seemed to say with infinite weariness, fatalistically. *And that's the way it's going to be.*

There seemed no reason for the dog to die after a week of intensive care; all my laboratory data showed that the collie was actually responding to my treatment. He *should* have been better. There was no longer any logical reason why he wasn't well by now—but he wasn't.

Late one night, as I stood looking into the cage, I suddenly felt a terrible fury welling up inside me. We'd been carrying this 120-pound urinating, defecating, rank hulk of a collie around for a week. He hadn't even made an effort to stand by himself. He didn't seem able to. Weary and beaten, I grew furious—and finally lost my temper! I marched into the cage, shouted, "You have absolutely no right to be lying in there sick," and impulsively booted Weepy in the rump.

To my astonishment, the dog leaped up and ran out to the front door. I couldn't believe my eyes. He hadn't seemed able to stand!

The next day the collie went home, perfectly fit, with a grateful family who considered me no less than a miracle worker.

That was many years ago. I haven't kicked a dog since then and never will, but only recently, thinking back over the case, did I suspect that this dog was winning his game by dying. If he had died, he would have proven to the world that he was really, truly sick. Until he finally realized, by virtue of the boot, that my office wasn't a fun place to play "Sick and Dying," he was intent on maintaining his scheme. There is no other plausible explanation. That kick, delivered in anger, was my most therapeutic gesture. Thereafter, I saw Weepy for the usual minor illnesses and as soon as he saw I had my shoes on, he got better fast.

At the time I had no idea what had happened. It was a curious incident. I was delighted the dog hadn't died, but whenever I thought about it, I had to laugh. Cured by a boot!

Some time later a psychiatrist brought in a rather high-strung cocker spaniel with hemorrhagic bowel movements. The dog was admitted to my hospital that evening, and I promptly gave him some medication. He responded by the next day. My treatment had been minimal, but the improvement was dramatic. To be sure, I kept the dog an extra day, spent a bit of time playing with him when I had a chance, and gave him special attention. Corky was a delightful dog, and I took a personal liking to him.

A few days after the psychiatrist took the dog home, he called me, furious. The dog had the same problem again.

Well, perhaps I hadn't treated him long enough; I thought I'd made that mistake before. When the owner brought him back again late that night, the dog looked an absolute wreck. I put him in the kennel again, but considering the hour, I decided to examine him the next day. The next morning the dog's bowel movement was perfectly normal.

To be certain the dog was really well this time, I kept him in the hospital another four or five days, watching him carefully, regulating his diet, paying him a great deal of attention but administering no medication, since none now seemed called for. Finally, when I was *positive* there could be no recurrence, I phoned the owner, and he came to my office that afternoon. In the waiting room on the way out, the dog suddenly stopped, hunched over—and there was the problem again.

After a while, I began to suspect a pattern; these animals were getting what they wanted by being in the hospital. Here they had regular contact with people; here they were the center of attention.

My interest in this odd phenomenon was piqued when I realized that an abnormally large number of dogs and cats brought in for routine spaying—generally an uneventful surgical procedure—would go home and promptly become sick.

"What did you do to my dog?" an owner would shout, so irate that the phone shook. The dog would be vomiting or twitching. A whole host of maladies would suddenly appear. But when I examined the animals, I could find no organic disturbances.

After a while, I began to suspect a pattern; these animals were getting what they wanted by being in the hospital. Here they had regular contact with people; here they were the center of attention. They were looked at, played with, coddled, and talked to. They must love it, I thought, and I remembered boyhood friends of mine who used to get sick a lot and then get chicken soup and sympathy and even presents from their mothers. These boys would stay sick.

In a similar way, the pets would go home and their owners would make a fuss over them for a day or so and then the excitement was abruptly over. Did the animals, finding themselves in an emotional vacuum, elect to play a sick game to regain the attention they missed?

Though I strongly suspected they did, at the time this idea sounded like an absurdity.

But postsurgical cases were becoming a real problem, and I kept brooding about them. At one time I would have thought that something had gone wrong with my treatment, but I began to feel more and more that something had gone too right. The animals had been treated with exceptional love and affection—and it didn't work.

The situation was a marvelous paradox, but I was faced with a sticky problem. Owners don't want to hear that their little pussy Trumpkin prefers the hospital to his home. "That cat is sick," they insist. "You must have fed him some poisonous food. Someone must have beaten him." One woman was so livid when I hinted at the real reason her cat had begun to vomit that she called me "a downright liar" and vanished from my practice forever. Had I told her that Pussy-boots had "eucalyptus of the blowhole, a frequent complication following spaying," and provided a cryptic prescription for an antibiotic, she'd still be bringing her seven cats to me every other week. I lost a small fortune when I was honest with her.

Finally, I decided to call a conference in my hospital. I gathered my six assistants together and said, "Listen. There's something going wrong here—and it's got to stop." Everyone looked at me and began to fidget.

"You guys," I said, looking at each of them intently, "are being too nice to the patients." Several of them began to smile.

"You have got to stop coddling the animals during post-operative care. I don't want you walking around holding these cats in your arms and playing Poor Baby with them. I don't want you petting the dogs or spending too much time with them. Understand? You're creating a tremendous problem for me."

By now they were all laughing—and I had to laugh with them. But it was a real problem.

I had finally, after many years, made my hospital precisely what I wanted it to be. I had enough assistants, and I was giving all the animals the ultimate in care. I could ask, "Did that dog eat? When was its last bowel movement?" and get accurate answers. I'd always wanted this kind of detailed information; it enabled me to take total responsibility in my treatment and care.

My hospital was functioning beautifully. But the system didn't work.

Instead of helping, I was deterring the animals' recovery. I was even losing clients because of the problem. I remembered then the dying collie I'd booted in the rump so many years before and the high-strung cocker spaniel with strangely recurrent bowel-movement problems. I decided firmly that the animals must get what they needed in my hospital and not one drop more.

No sooner did I put this system into effect than the incidence of postoperative "disease" declined sharply. Some animals still wanted to come back; some still seemed intent on proving their point by threatening to die. According to their situations, they all got exactly what they needed and nothing more.

I suppose I am even rougher on them in my office today. "Listen," I tell many of them, "I want you up and out of here pronto. I want none of your games." I might scare them, but I let the animals know they will get the treatment they need but no pampering. "Out," I say when I need to. "You're cured. I know it, and you know it. No more games."

> *The art of postoperative care—or noncare—is the art of blending just enough of Poor Baby with just enough of "Kick in the Rump."*

I've seen dozens of animals quickly find the will to get out; I've seen several stagger to their feet and head toward the door. They get the point. They know I know. Several even seem to say sheepishly, *Oh, darn.*

*I can't bluff this guy for a minute. He knows what games I'm
playing, and it won't be fun here at all. I might as well trudge
home.*

Animals now get the best possible treatment in my
"Intensive-I-Don't-Care Unit." They are out of my hospital a
lot quicker than they would be out of most other hospitals,
they recover faster, and I have done a lot less. Truly, I have
become an expert in postoperative nursing and how important it is not.

Outside the hospital, I have seen many animals playing
the same game. I have owned several myself. Mordecai the
goat was a particularly subtle offender, and I, like everyone
else, usually fell into his trap. One night the little goat
became colicky and screamed so much that the next morning I was afraid to leave him at home. So I put him into the
car and headed off for work, thinking I could treat him better
in my office.

My secretary—who had magnificent mothering tenden-
cies—held that adorable baby goat in her arms all day.
People in the waiting room made a fuss over the animal all

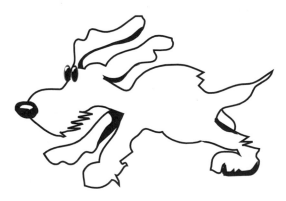

day as my secretary
played an extravagant
game of Poor Baby. I
had a chance to
examine the animal
briefly and found
nothing wrong. By the
end of the day the
goat was fine, and
when I got him home he ran vigorously into the pen.

But the next morning he was sick again, vomiting and weak-kneed. His bleats were nearly heartrending, but not quite. I examined him closely and then said, "No way. Not today. Get better right where you are—not on my secretary's lap, where I know you'd like to be."

The goat made an uneventful recovery without treatment.

The rules of good postoperative care are simple. Pets like to be cuddled. People like to cuddle pets. Cuddling pets when they're sick or recovering from an illness only encourages them to remain sick. The art of postoperative care—or noncare—is the art of blending just enough of Poor Baby with just enough of "Kick in the Rump."

CHAPTER 13

Nontreatment Treatments and the Ultimate Placebo

TWO WOMEN CAME TO MY OFFICE with a cat. One of the women, the owner, was in her twenties. The other, a neighbor and cat maven, was slightly older and much more sophisticated. The cat was suffering from a severe case of conjunctivitis. It was a real disease—the eyes were discharging pus, there was extreme redness around the lids, and the cat was clearly suffering from painful sensitivity to light. Conjunctivitis happens to be a common disease among cats.

The cat maven promptly took charge and told me they'd taken the animal to several veterinarians, who had prescribed various eye drops to be administered regularly or when the cat was in particular discomfort. Nothing had helped. The eyes had remained virtually the same, and the women now wanted my help.

I examined the cat carefully, then asked the owner, "Do you clean his eyes out every morning when you get up?"

"Yes. I dab them with cotton, too, whenever he rubs and I see the pus. And I give him medicine and drops three times a day."

"Does the cat like being given the drops?"

"Absolutely not! I have to chase him all over the house. Prudence," she added, nodding to her friend the cat maven, "insists that I do it religiously, no matter how much trouble it takes; so I stop whatever I happen to be doing and take care of him."

"Fine," I said. "Now let's play a game. Here's some cotton. Every time I rub my eyes, like this, will you agree to come over, look closely at them, and then dab them with this piece of cotton?"

The owner giggled, as people usually do when I put them through this routine; the cat maven frowned.

"You agree to do it every time, okay?"

Now they both frowned. The owner looked a little embarrassed. Prudence, the cat maven, was becoming bored, but the owner reluctantly agreed to play the game. I rubbed my eyes, and she came over, then hesitated; it was too ridiculous.

"You agreed," I insisted.

"Must I?" she asked.

"This is silly," Prudence said.

"She has no choice," I said. "She agreed to do it every time."

"Oh, all right," the owner said. She came over, took my head in the crook of her arm, and then rubbed first my left, then my right eye gently with the cotton. It felt rather good.

We repeated the game three times, and I said, "Great. You're getting the signals and performing right on cue. But see how I'm running your life?"

The owner started to laugh, but Prudence said, "You *have* to be kidding."

"Nope. That's what's going on here."

"I can understand," Prudence said, "how some things are psychosomatic, but you can't seriously want us to believe that's the case here. Look at the pus. Can pus be formed by the brain?"

The pus was quite real, as real as any symptom. I assured her the body does what the mind tells it to do. In spite of the pus, the cat was playing a game and the owner was abetting him.

> *I assured her the body does what the mind tells it to do . . . the cat was playing a game and the owner was abetting him.*

"I don't buy that for one minute," the cat maven said, shaking her head.

I took a chance and told them exactly how I read the situation: the cat was indeed playing a game. I told them the cat probably said something like this: I *think I'll give her the signal. I'll rub my eyes, and then she'll chase me all over the house and under the bed. Then she'll get down on her hands and knees. What a fun game!*

I advised the women that I could treat the conjunctivitis classically—as the other veterinarians had done without result. Or we could try something else.

The owner, at least, was willing to try something else.

So I got out an empty dropper bottle and told the owner to fill it three-quarters full of water. "Then," I said, my voice taking on the edge of the old authoritative doctor, "you add two drops of your smelliest perfume, shake, and apply three times a day or whenever you find the cat in particular discomfort. Make a ceremony of taking the bottle out and rubbing it into . . . "

"Not his *eyes!*" said Prudence, shocked. "You can't *mean* it."

"Not for a minute," I said. "Rub the solution into the base of his *tail*—very ceremoniously. Then maybe the cat will say to himself, *Oh, so that's where it's at now! It's* not *the eyes any more. It's back there!* I'll bet the conjunctivitis clears up promptly."

This time the maven was certain I was crazy. But the owner had already spent a great deal of time and money on other veterinarians and medications and this "medicine" of mine cost only a nickel for the bottle, so she was a good sport. "Oh, what can I lose, Pru?" she asked, laughing.

A week later she called to tell me that Fluffy's "eye disease" was completely cured.

After some time I expanded the application of this brilliant cure. I began to treat ear infections, a common complaint, with oil of clove on the base of the tail. There are a lot of spicy-smelling dogs around whose ears have cleared up spontaneously.

Many people will do anything possible to avoid being uncomfortable, and for such people—as you saw in chapter 11, which discussed pain—nothing is more uncomfortable than seeing their pet uncomfortable. They are chronic pill dispensers. They put infinite trust in the tools of modern science. Put such a person together with a new intern, anxious to cure everything in sight by classical methods, and you can support a dozen drug companies. Nothing, I suspect, is more dangerous to the ultimate well-being of pet, owner, or even doctor. The pet may get stuck in its belief that being sick is winning the game, the owner will never get to experience suppressed feelings to completion because he or she will always be looking for painkillers and cure-alls, and the doctor will not really be healing, only repairing faulty plumbing. Playing "Hearts and Flowers" on the violin, which I told one woman to do when her cat started to whine, is more effective.

> *I eventually resorted more and more often to a magic cure—old Dr. Tanzer's occult, remarkable, unfailing "Superfixiola"— nothing.*

In fact, I eventually resorted more and more often to a magic cure—old Dr. Tanzer's occult, remarkable, unfailing "Superfixiola"—*nothing*.

"What should we *doooo?*" owners ask plaintively.

"Nothing," I tell them, knowing how hard it will be for them to stick to this prescription.

"When you call me in a week, I'm going to ask you, 'How is the twitching?'" I tell an owner for whose pet I had just prescribed nothing. "What are you going to tell me?"

"I hope," she says timidly, "that I'll be able to tell you he's better."

"No, no, no, no!" I shout. "You have to do *nothing*. If you look, that's *something*. You're looking—and that's precisely what the little con artist wants."

"Oh," the owner says sheepishly.

"There's only one answer I can possibly accept: I don't know."

Though nothing is often an extremely effective medicine, "nothing with a flair" is often even a bit better.

One woman brought in a dachshund with a history of disk disease, spinal problems accompanied by periodic pain. I asked her about the dog's back while I was giving him a routine check-up last June before she went on her summer holiday. "Oh, it's been fine," she said. "It flares up every few days—I can see him favoring his back and in pain—but I just give him an aspirin and in ten minutes he's better."

I thought about suggesting to her that it's impossible for aspirin to dissipate a dog's back pain in ten minutes, but I sensed it would be futile. I did not want to push the issue, but I did not want that dog taking aspirin, either. So I told her I'd gotten a new drug in. It was much more potent than aspirin and much safer. "Try it," I said. "If it works, it's much better for the dog."

In the other room I took out a pill envelope and poured twenty or thirty Tic Tac mints into it.

A month later, when she returned to the city, she called to say they'd worked beautifully; in fact, she wanted more.

Six months later the dog was still responding well to these miracle pills. What the dog really wanted was the physical act of getting the pill. This act made the dog feel a connection to the owner. When your Mommy puts her hand halfway down your throat, you know you exist.

Unfortunately, I couldn't tell the woman the truth. She had to believe in the pills or they might stop working.

One of the most interesting instances of the potency of placebos is the "Cocktail-Frankfurter Case."

A pleasant couple, an older man and woman, brought in a crossbred basset-fox terrier, a funny, little short-coated dog with small, pigeon-toed legs and a face with a black eye that was right out of the *Our Gang* comedies. He looked as if they'd put the wrong parts together in making him. I loved the dog immediately.

The dog had a history of prostatitis and had been passing blood in his urine. I examined him carefully, finally passing a catheter into him and finding no obstruction that might require surgery. Based on the symptoms—high frequency of urination, pain while urinating, the presence of blood—I made the diagnosis of a bladder infection.

The man wanted to know what caused this, and I told him—right out of the textbook, because that seemed to be what he wanted—that older dogs like this one frequently got bacterial infections of this sort. When the prostate became a bit enlarged around the neck of the bladder, there was some retention of urine, which caused bacteria to grow and infection to set in.

"Neck of the bladder . . . bacteria . . . " he said, nodding. The terms were properly technical and gave a logical cause he could live with. He felt safe with the facts. "Well," he said, "what do we do about it?"

I advised him that I'd give the dog an injection to help flush out his bladder and dilute the urine. With medication, the dog would be better within about ten days.

As I injected the dog and watched him on the table, taking the full thrust of the needle without flinching, I began to suspect old Black Eye was saying, *Oh, thank you for all that pain. I really love it, Doc. A little more, please, so those good people will pet me nice and proper when we get home. It's great. You don't know the kind of attention they're giving me. And being here on the table? Usually human beings are at the table and I'm on the floor. I've really made it! All these people, so concerned about me!*

I even thought I saw the old faker wink at me.

The people went home, and the dog's problems cleared up shortly. When I was a new vet-school graduate I would

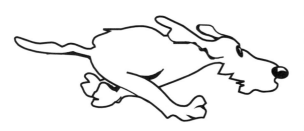

have felt completely validated by this experience. "They told me if I use these particular pills, I can cure

such urinary infections—and that's what happened."

I suspected otherwise.

Something—whether grandchildren came to visit or the walls were painted (I never learned)—had threatened the dog. He'd gone back to the birth experience, which involved fear for survival, and he remembered how his mother had licked his genitalia and stimulated him to urinate. Urinating a lot, as often as possible, was clearly linked with survival. The dog had started to urinate frequently. And then—and this is the important fact in this case—Mommy and Daddy gave him all the attention he needed. He was convinced he'd found the right tape. And his owners got a chance to feel sorry, to play "Worried Owner." They were nice folks and clearly liked the game.

When I'd told them the dog was all right, when I'd given them a medical cause, they were relieved, and they stopped worrying so much. But the dog wasn't cured. Two weeks later, more worried than ever, they brought that funny, little black eyed dog in with the same symptoms.

I took x-rays this time, checked the dog again thoroughly, and finally said, "I still don't think this is anything to worry about. Keep him on those pills for three more weeks."

The woman protested. "But doctor, it was extremely difficult to give him the pills."

I began to suggest that the dog really liked the no doubt elaborate ritual of pill taking, but the man interrupted: "Absolutely not. He hated to take the medicine."

"Really?" I asked, feeling that I had my foot in the door, that I was beginning to understand the problem. "Do you chase him around?"

"We did for the first week, but we had to follow him all over the house. He'd go under the bed, and we'd drag him out and hold him and shove the pills down."

The old "Take-the-Pill Game," I thought. What attention! What fun! I began to tell them, but the man interrupted again.

"Then," he said, "we decided to use little cocktail frankfurters. You see, we slit the frankfurters, put the pill inside, and he took it quite well. We did that three times a day until the ten days were up."

That was it. Old Black Eye positively loved cocktail frankfurters, three times a day, given to him by Mommy and Daddy.

I prescribed the same pills for another two weeks, administered in cocktail frankfurters. "Then," I said, "I want you to give the dog just cocktail frankfurters, without pills, for another two weeks."

The good people looked at me as if I were definitely mad. They were speechless.

"Look. There's an outside chance that the dog is a first-rate con man and gets himself sick just to get the franks."

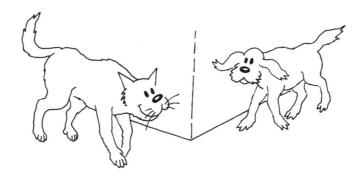

They laughed, and I did, too. Laughter is healthy.

"It's less expensive," I said, "and less involved than bringing the dog in for removal of his prostate. I don't think he needs it. What have we got to lose?"

So we put him on the regimen, and the dog has stayed symptom-free since—on cocktail frankfurters three times a day.

The ultimate placebo, then, is nothing given with a flair.

This prescription isn't good for me, the doctor, or for the drug company. But it's great for the old dog, who loves franks, and for Armour, the company that makes them.

The two concerned owners could find worse things to do than feed Black Eye cocktail frankfurters every day and laugh with their neighbors about it all.

Only sometimes I wonder what will happen when the news of this cure gets out. Will someone get a $2 million grant to figure out what ingredient in cocktail franks cures bladder infections?

CHAPTER 14

Multiple Pets

WHEN THERE ARE SEVERAL PETS in one family, the game playing gets complicated. The pets often take on particular roles,
according to when they were acquired, their size, and how they are
treated by the human beings. They may establish "sibling" rivalries
and vie for an owner's attention, or they may place themselves on
the sphere and identify themselves in relation to the other pets.

One owner has a cat and a dog. The cat nurses the dog, and it's
obvious her favorite game is Poor Baby. There's usually a "victim" in
every menagerie, a good guy who waits with apparently infinite
patience and charity until everyone else is finished at the food dish.
Mommy always worries her little heart out about Schlump. "He's
such a good cat. Why does he let the others take such unfair advantage of him all the time? But Mommy loves him, doesn't she?" she
says as she cuddles, him tenderly. Schlump is winning with his act.
He's discovered that one way to be successful is to appear as if he's
not.

One family with a Doberman pinscher, a dachshund, and several cats, discovered that the Doberman, the largest and presumably strongest animal of the group, gets sick most often. I questioned the grown daughter, who brought the dog in, and she told me that the smaller animals seem to get more of the natural sympathy in the family. So the Doberman gets sick, really sick. You can see by her pathetic facial expression that she is Suzy Sick. You can see she's always suffering so much and that it's all so painful.

I treated her diarrhea successfully, but three days later she started act 2: urinating in the kitchen. And then a week later, she went lame.

She stood in my office with that terribly sore and painful front right leg, and I asked her in my throatiest Marlene Dietrich voice, "What's the matter this time, sweetheart?"

She came hobbling over to me and, with that Suzy Sick look on her face, picked up her front leg for me to examine.

I'd already told the daughter what was going on, and when the Doberman came over and showed me her problem, we both laughed openly.

Suzy Sick, her eyes embarrassed but still full of self-pity, said, *What can I do? It's the only way they'll pay attention to an awesome-looking creature like poor me.*

One family with two dogs, male and female adults, brought the female in with a messy problem: she had developed an overpowering scent. Odors have always been great survival mechanisms for dogs; it is hard not to be noticed when you stink. Some of the foulest-smelling dogs I know—absolute sewers!—are some of the happiest: *everyone* knows they're there.

This dog's problem was immediately apparent; her vagina was badly inflamed. The owner had tried three veterinarians at considerable expense. None had been able to produce a cure.

I examined the dog and then began my questioning. I asked when the owner had first noticed the odor.

She couldn't remember.

I insisted she try harder. She certainly could remember when an odor like this one started.

"Well, it was *about* the time the cat died," she said.

"Did the dog *like* the cat?" I asked.

"Hardly! She never stopped nipping and barking, chasing the cat around the house, under the beds, into the kitchen, behind the couch."

Odors have always been great survival mechanisms for dogs; it is hard not to be noticed when you stink. Some of the foulest-smelling dogs I know—absolute sewers!—are some of the happiest: everyone knows they're there.

Her answers interested me. We talked more. I suspected before long that the dog had felt an immense loss when the cat died. It was also possible that when the cat was gone, the dog simply needed something to do. Boredom is a notorious producer of mischief in pets—and in human beings, too. The inflammation had been caused by intense licking of the vulva. The dog had started this soon after the cat died, probably because she felt she wouldn't survive without her feline friend. It was the fear-for-survival, recollection-of-the-birth-experience pattern again. She had remembered her mother's tongue licking her at another time when her survival was threatened. But what had caused the problem to become so serious?

The initial licking felt good, so she did more of it. Since survival is a desperate business, she then began to lick furiously. This caused an inflammation and some odor. The odor then attracted the male dog, who came over and also began licking the spayed female (spaying would normally have short-circuited a male's interest). *This game is getting better and better,* the dog must have thought. The female grew more and more fixated on her genital area; she began to lick frantically. The male became more interested, and he too began to lick harder. The owner then became terribly upset at the increasingly rank odor and began to play Poor Baby with the female and look closely at the inflamed area a dozen times a day. The male dog and the owner succeeded in giving the female dog more attention than she'd ever had in her life.

Far out! she thought. *It works. This is heaven . . . only it's beginning to hurt a little down there.*

From the dog's point of view, the worst thing I could have done would have been to cure her. She didn't want to get better. And my own actions to this point hadn't been any help. I'd merely given the affected area *more* attention in the format of a doctor with scrubbed gloves, a nurse, and an attendant all standing around the table, with the attendant holding a spotlight close to the inflamed vulva.

> *From the dog's point of view, the worst thing I could have done would have been to cure her. She didn't want to get better.*

Terrific, the dog thought. *It's a little scary—but boy, am I surviving! What next?*

Standard medical practice in a case as bad as this one would be to require at least a week's stay in the hospital. The area would have to be shaved and carefully medicated. Plastic surgery might be required on either side of the vulva. In such a case, the dog might well end up thinking, *This hurts so much, I'm giving up this game.* Then again she might not.

The other way to treat her would be to explain the problem to the owners as clearly as possible and to suggest a cure that would address the issue at its root. After some discussion, this is what I decided to do. Happily, they found my ideas not ludicrous but fascinating. But what, precisely, could they do?

Vaginal licking with such fury happens to be a potentially bad game. Many dogs simply get too much from the act in too many ways and won't give it up. In this case multiple pets complicated the issue. Even if the female stopped licking, might not the male continue?

I recommended two things: separate the male dog from the female for an extended period of time and despite the odor, stop paying the female special attention when she licks. I knew the chief danger: the odor might become so intense that the people simply would not (and should not) tolerate it any more. The dog might then have to be hospitalized or even destroyed.

Fortunately, this did not happen. I administered steroids, which gave the dog a sufficient feeling of euphoria, so she did not need to lick. The owners boarded out the male dog for a month. They also did an excellent job of holding their noses (when the dog couldn't see) and doing nothing, and the pattern was broken.

The second dog complicated this particular case, but in most families, like mine, multiple pets distinctly add to the joy of owning animals. Most of the games they play with one another are harmless—and often fascinating to watch.

While my children were growing up, I began to collect a huge, happy menagerie of pets. Besides Hildy, the zoo at its largest was composed of four goats, a parrot, a macaw, approximately fifteen rabbits, nine cats, three kittens, three horses, about two million honey bees, Elmo the one-eyed English fighting cock, and Loony, a young raccoon. Elmo, who is seventeen years old, has a speech impediment that makes his crow sound like a scratchy phonograph. He sleeps on a divider between the box stalls in the barn where the wild raccoons can't get him, and he doesn't crow on Sundays until 9:00 A.M., except when he becomes confused and crows at 2:30 A.M.

They have all been a great joy to me with their respective games, and since the pets are constantly reproducing, I have had the repeated and exciting experience of creation taking place all around me. One of my goats once gave birth during our Passover dinner—hence the name Mordecai for the game-playing kid. Another goat began to fail one evening, and I can remember bringing it to the dinner table and listening to it *baa-ah* and bleat and then revive in time for us to finish our meal. My family's life has always revolved around animals; once we even made space in our family room for a diamondback rattlesnake.

Our animal society is clearly composed of potential combatants. Roosters and raccoons are considered natural enemies; birds and cats and cats and dogs are not supposed to get along together. Dogs seem to *know* they're expected to chase cats, but chasing cats was not expected in my house.

I let all the animals know, "If you guys want to kill one another, go ahead; if you want to live here together, great." They seemed to get the point.

When my oldest daughter brought Elmo home, I turned him loose in the barnyard despite some fears that the cats would catch him. They caught wild birds all the time. I watched one of our black cats come stalking up close and eye the rooster. I didn't say a word, but I knew that old Elmo looked like a delicious dinner. The cat looked at Elmo, Elmo looked at the cat, and both were tense for a moment. Then the cat relaxed and turned away, saying, *Oh. He lives here. Elmo's okay.*

Elmo, who sleeps in our horse Scrumpy's stall, defecates on Scrumpy regularly—and the horse feels that this is an expression of love like sending flowers.

The interaction is fascinating to watch. When we remove all our human interference and our so-called sophistication, everyone seems to let everyone else be, which is the way it should be.

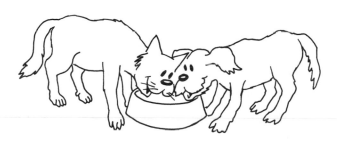

When Loony, the raccoon, came, he looked at the horses, the cats looked at him, he looked at Elmo, and before long they were all old chums.

Of course there are rituals as in any society. Stanley, my son's horse, seems to play a particular role in this world. His role is "Chief Stomper." He seems to step on everyone. At last count he's managed to step on my foot, Elmo's tailfeathers—so we ended up with a bare-rumped fighting cock—and most recently, Loony's paw. He's also broken three of Hildy's ribs. Stanley welcomes new creatures into the Tanzer family by stepping on them; if they survive Stanley, they are welcome to live here.

Having so many pets complicates our lives tremendously. At times it is a madhouse. But we choose that way and enjoy the fun. If we didn't enjoy it, we'd get rid of the animals.

Other owners, I fear, don't choose. They feel they must adopt more and more pets, as I showed earlier, in chapter 4. They don't enjoy their pets, since they feel forced by their own fear of abandonment to create so many. I know one woman with 123 adopted cats. Her little home smells like one gigantic litter box. And think of the money she spends buying cat food!

Some of these chronic adopters suddenly come to a realization and say, "Oh, it's not that I *like* pets so much; I just *hate* abandonment." So they create a philanthropic organization called "Spay Your Little Puppies" or "Hysterectomies Galore" or "Everybody's Ovaries Out," to obliterate abandonment from the universe. These organizations may do some good for the animals in the community, but they won't work any better than the 123 cats to make chronic adopters feel complete. These "antiabandonmentarians" will simply have to recognize, one day, that they feel as though they themselves were abandoned, have a good long cry, and complete the feelings of abandonment in their own lives (basically, get over it).

Multiple pets should bring joy, but *more* won't prove to be better, if they've been brought home for the wrong reasons.

CHAPTER 15

Hildy and Me

ONE MORNING MY WIFE AND I PREPARED to leave home and head for my hospital. One of my secretaries was ill, and my wife was going to help me for a few days. As we got ready and gave a few last instructions to the children, I noticed that Hildy was acting strangely—pawing, whining a bit, moving about restlessly. That didn't surprise me because Hildy often acts strangely. She has a thousand games.

That morning she sensed something was different. My wife and I were *both* leaving. The children would soon be going to school. Poor Hildy would be alone.

As we were about to leave, poor Hildy suddenly came up to us with a vastly sad look in her eye and a *pincushion* in her mouth as if to say, *Look. If you two leave, I'll just kill myself. I swear. I'll kill myself with these pins.*

What could we do? We *had* to take her with us.

We spoiled the dog terribly. She is not allowed at the dinner table—except at mealtimes. She is a finicky eater and often won't touch a speck of prepared dog food. But she'll steal half a coconut custard pie out of the kitchen, then come in sheepishly to confess her sins. What can we do?

Once she was lost for an afternoon, and in a panic, we called the police. But that evening she came sauntering back, carrying a lunch bag that she'd stolen from a workman.

The horses have their games, too. We had trouble getting Stanley, one of our stallions, into the trailer one day, but when our son's mare, Scrumpy was led in, Stanley followed eagerly. Jackson, a stallion who never likes to get into the trailer, put his feet up on the back of the trailer and began to cry and whinny and beg to be let in. Scrumpy once stayed lame for eight weeks, and I got so caught up in her game and felt so sorry for her, that I had x-rays taken and a special shoe made. But we couldn't find a thing wrong organically. Then one day I'd had enough of the game, so I got out her saddle. My son Kenny jogged her around the paddock. She was still as lame as ever. I walked up to her with a pot of glue in hand, confronted her, and said, "So, Scrumpy, still lame, huh? Well, see this?" I raised the pot, so it was inches from her eye. "See this glue pot, Scrumpy? You could be in there. You're cured, and I want you to cut out this nonsense."

Whereupon my son took her out, rode her all afternoon, and didn't notice then or afterward a touch of lameness.

As long as I felt sorry for her, as long as I was concerned and caring and making a fuss over her, she stayed sick—just as you or I would and every animal does. When I stopped, she stopped.

I have a close-up photograph of Hildy on my office wall; her big sleepy head is nestled in comfort on the couch (from which she is theoretically banned). I regularly point out the photo to patients, especially when they are convinced that they have the only pet in the world who plays outrageous games with his or her owner. I have such a pet, too, the photo says. And I am a bigger sucker than they are. It is humiliating that even though my pets have a veterinarian for an owner—someone who *knows*—they still get away with most of their games.

Pincushions, indeed!

If there is a "Tanzer Method," surely it should include the *right* way to handle a pet. Just as surely, if there is a right way, I should use it with Hildy.

I'm quite definitely human, and Hildy constantly trains me and makes me the fall guy. Frankly, I wouldn't have it any other way. I don't want to master or control the dog but to live with her as closely as possible. Knowledge is essential because if I know the games Hildy is playing and recognize the fact that I am causing her to play them, I can enjoy the games rather than be a slave to them. My most practical advice to pet owners is this: *be more conscious.* And then, as the cases in this book have shown, once you

> *It is humiliating that even though my pets have a veterinarian for an owner—someone who knows—they still get away with most of their games.*

recognize the cause of the problems, they will vanish if you want them to.

I love Hildy and let her be what she is—an incredibly human, mischievous hunk of a dog, involved in a perpetual theatrical production in which she plays a score of roles. Also, I am quite willing to admit that I am just like Hildy.

Why do I tolerate Hildy laying waste to half a coconut custard pie, snoozing on the furniture, threatening me with pincushions? Because I do the same kinds of things, and I'd like the world to tolerate me the way I tolerate Hildy.

I never experienced my string of yappy Yorkshire terriers the way I experience this dog. I know I didn't acquire Hildy; I *created* her. I wanted a big, robust dog. Our physical structure is similarly stocky, muscular, even brutish. Our eyes are so much the same color and shape, I often feel as though I am looking into a mirror. Hildy's upper teeth are perfect, her lowers misaligned. So are mine. She's a compulsive eater and, I have to admit, I am, too.

The dog has always caused some pain in her world—playing hard, biting hard—but nothing very serious. She is slightly destructive but never with anything that really matters.

Looking at Hildy, I can see myself and can thus *use* myself to better advantage, because watching her gives me insight about myself and how I look to the rest of the world. I must be frightening to some people because of the way I look, I often think, Let me play up my softness—and perhaps, when the situation warrants, like on a subway late at night, *use* my ominous exterior.

My children experience Hildy as soft, fun to play with, but sometimes a nuisance. Do they see me that way too?

How does Hildy fit into my wife's life? How does Hildy relate to new friends? To the universe? There's so much I can learn from that dog. She is a magnificent working model of me for me to observe.

One afternoon, I brought home a pound of cashews, put them on the living room table, and went in to sit at the kitchen table with the rest of my family. Hildy, a compulsive eater, walked into the living room, saw the cashews sitting on the table, no doubt said, *Hang it, I'm going to eat them all,* and promptly did.

A few minutes later, my wife discovered the tragedy, came rushing in, and announced that every one of the nuts was gone.

Whereupon Hildy, a tank of a dog, came slowly in, her ears back, saying, *Oh, I'm terribly sorry I did this, but*

Whereupon David, my oldest son, a vegetarian perfectly mad for cashews, slapped Hildy in the head. Hildy took it calmly, as if it was part of the deal.

Whereupon my good wife, so soft of heart, rushed to the rescue saying, "Don't hit her for that!"

"Are you kidding?" David retorted.

What a game! Everybody played and everybody won.

Hildy got a full stomach and a chance to be the "Sorrowful Offender" and the "Slap Victim." My son played "Offended Victim" in this particular drama. My wife played the "Compassionate Mother" in her usual game of Poor Baby. The rest of my children took sides and positions, which they love to do. And I, the doctor, watched this fascinating little game *in my own home,* of all places, and laughed.

Laughter, as I said, is healthy.

Perhaps this is the best practical advice of all: be able to see the game, identify it for what it is, know who's who and what the payoff is, and laugh.

Perhaps this is the best practical advice of all: be able to see the game, identify it for what it is, know who's who and what the payoff is, and laugh.

I may have all this remarkable clarity about pet games, but I still have to keep telling myself some day I won't let Hildy get away with so much.

Pincushions!

CHAPTER 16

The Sex Game

SEX, FOR PETS AS WELL AS HUMAN BEINGS, is a highly serious matter. It can also be hilarious or absurd.

The female dog or cat will accept a mate only when she is able to reproduce, and at such time, she will accept practically any handy male. There is conspicuously little matching of size in dogs. A female dog in heat will say brazenly, *Take me,* and a male dog, sometimes four times her size and sometimes a quarter of it, will charge like a bull and experience incredible discomfort trying to find a way to comply. Male dogs are *always* interested. Whenever Hildy is in heat, there are lots of assorted males—of all different sizes and shapes and breeds, some of whom make treacherous journeys from miles away—camped out on our doorstep and capable of waiting endlessly for an opportunity with my gorgeous bull mastiff.

Female cats will not ovulate until they actually have sexual relations. The male cat's penis has barbs on it, and thus neither male nor female wants to—or really can—separate before ejaculation. Such perfect timing and what might be called a "fertility hook" explain why there are so many cats in the world. We have had twelve. Or is it thirteen?

The male dog has a bulb at the base of his penis, and the female's vagina will constrict around this, locking the mating pair together. This explains why we see so many dogs stuck together.

A boar will spend an afternoon twisting his corkscrew penis into the proper circuit. This lengthy process surely encourages fertilization.

And the queen bee will keep a small tribe of male drones like gigolos, whose sole function is to mate with her. Though she only mates once, the males stay in the hive, never go out to work, and are fed and catered to by the workers. In winter, when the productive season is over and there is a need to conserve food, the drones are summarily thrown out to be killed by the cold. Every fall I have seen this shocking drama in my own hives.

Human beings *think* more about sex and have expanded the game in subtlety, variety, and selectivity. We like our lives to be complicated, so we demand an elaborate mating ritual. Animals are indifferent to these human niceties, and this indifference is especially evident when pets masturbate. *They* haven't been told it will cause cancer or pimples; they don't know they should take cold showers instead. Many dogs, particularly males, who are always ready, will mount an owner's leg anywhere and anytime. Dogs who have been raised with people, not other dogs, often develop sexual as well as emotional attachments to human beings.

I have had literally hundreds of owners come to me, show me some insignificant scratch that was the pretext under which they made an appointment, and then in a voice filled with flagrant embarrassment say, "Also . . . Max is . . . uh . . . well . . .

"You mean, he's *masturbating?*"

"Well . . . uh . . . yes. That's right. He's doing it." And in a frantic tone they ask, "All the time. *Everywhere!* What should I do?"

"What are you doing now?" I ask.

And then I hear the scenario begin to unfold. Whenever he masturbates, they lock him up, yank on his collar, beat him with a stick, or scream at him.

The problem started, I learned in one case, when the owner's charming elderly aunt, with a 1920s-style dress and curled white hair, came over for tea one afternoon. Smooch suddenly mounted the aunt's leg.

"What did you do?" I asked.

"Whaddaya *think* I did?" The owner is suddenly outraged at my innocence. "I socked the mutt!" Nobody masturbates in *his* house.

So Smooch, socked nearly senseless by his humiliated owner, ran under the table, shook and shivered for an hour until the aunt left, and then peeped out. The owner, by now feeling a bit bad about hitting the dog came over and said, "All right, Smooch. You didn't mean it. Come over here now and let me give you a hug."

That sock hurt a little, the dog thinks, *but I know Daddy still loves me—and that rubbing up and down sure was fun.*

Deep down the aunt was probably amused by this incident. The owner was embarrassed at first, but in the end he had a chance to show what an extraordinarily forgiving man he was. Despite the masturbating, he still loved Smooch, that is until Smooch did it again. In effect, that's what he'd been trained to do.

In another case, a spitz-beagle cross named Rex mounted a two-year-old child whom neighbors had brought over for a visit. I learned that the dog was probably afraid his owner was paying too much attention to this new little character in the play. His sudden fear for survival may have triggered a recollection of the birth experience when the mother licked his genitalia while he nursed. He sought to duplicate that original feeling in his genitalia—a feeling connected to survival. The dog had his attention caught by the child who was the center of attention, so he killed two birds with one stone. When he was shouted at and hit, he thought, *The right tape! This rubbing produces pleasure—and Daddy's sure proved he knows I'm still here.*

One fascinating case involved a woman who came in with her married daughter and a standard poodle with an earache. Mrs. Quigley, the mother, was elegant in both looks and actions. Her black couturier dress was exquisitely tailored to her trim figure and set off by a pearl necklace and earrings. Her husband was prosperous and influential. She'd been in my office many times before, and I liked her. Her poodle was also elegant. Othello stood very tall, and his jet

black, well-groomed trim made him a particularly handsome
specimen of a handsome breed.

While I was treating the ear infection, Mrs. Quigley
asked, without particular embarrassment, "By the way, what
can I do about this dog's masturbating? It's really a problem."

"Yes," the daughter added, "it genuinely is."

I asked them to tell me exactly what was going on.

Well, Mrs. Quigley apparently held a good number of
cocktail parties for her many friends, club members, and
political associates. "It happens mostly at the parties," she
explained. "The dog . . . well, mounts everybody who comes
in. Only last week Jane McBride was bending over the
punch bowl and . . . It's really quite embarrassing."

I could see how it might be.

I asked them to look at the situation objectively. Only the
animals who walk on two legs assign terms like "good" and
"bad" to such acts. To the dog,
sex of any kind was scarcely
"bad"; it was neither wrong nor
dirty. In fact, it was chiefly a way
he had of expressing his relatedness. When there was suddenly
an influx of potential playmates,
he wanted nothing more than to
experience being related to them.

"What do you do," I asked,
"when he does that?"

"We scold him."

"Ahhh. He's won both ways. He gets enjoyment out of
what he's doing sexually and then gets a bonus because

> To the dog, sex of any kind
> was scarcely "bad"; it was
> neither wrong nor dirty. In
> fact, it was chiefly a way
> he had of expressing his
> relatedness. When there
> was suddenly an influx of
> potential playmates, he
> wanted nothing more than
> to experience being
> related to them.

you single him out, point at him, and show him special attention. You're in fact training him to believe that masturbating is the right thing to do. Do you think he's going to give that up? No way. It feels terrific—and he gets your concern, too."

Mrs. Quigley began to smile and then chuckled.

Since I knew her well, I made a bold stab: "Tell me the truth, Mrs. Quigley. I sense that you're not really so concerned about all this, that in fact . . . "

"What are you talking about?" she asked, her voice a touch sharper.

"I can just picture one of your stuffy cocktail parties. One of the guests, in a short, elegant dress, bends over the onion dip with a potato chip and . . . I sense that you enjoy every minute of it, that sometimes you're so bored with the party and the people, you're glad it's happening."

This time she and her daughter laughed openly. A moment later Mrs. Quigley admitted that I was 100 percent correct.

Now, with the charged atmosphere gone and the game disclosed, we could begin to deal with the problem. Mrs. Quigley and I knew that no matter how natural her pet's act is, it's often inappropriate—socially unacceptable in our social world.

There are many ways to deal with acts of this kind. The most successful, always, is to do nothing. The dog will probably then say, *Nothing seems to be happening. Maybe I should chew up the Sunday* Times *instead.* The chances are that his position on that sphere I mentioned, his place in the household, is more important than the act itself.

Being able to talk about the situation and name it, as I did with Mrs. Quigley, is extremely important. At once everything begins to improve. Remember, the more you resist—mentally or physically—the more a problem will persist.

In a room full of people, though you may do nothing, there's little chance you'll get everyone else to go along with you. One outraged man may belt the dog; a woman may scream.

> *There are many ways to deal with acts of this kind. The most successful, always, is to do nothing.*

The dog can easily make himself the event of the evening. *Something* must be done.

Something drastic would be stepping on the dog's foot every time he gets up on someone—nothing else, no words, just that. Pretty soon the dog will say, *Wow, mounting someone feels good, but my foot sure doesn't. That feels bad more than the other feels good.*

Doing nothing may help the issue disappear in time, but you may need quicker results. Perhaps the most successful "treatment" is simply to take the dog away each time he masturbates when it is inappropriate and put him into the bathroom. The dog may be masturbating because he loves you or to get attention. Your solution may lie in providing, with an air of absolute certainty, the opposite. By silently picking him up, without display, and locking him away from people for an hour or so, you will make the dog think, *Every time I do this, I get ignored—just what I don't want. It isn't working.* You'll be removing him from yourself or other people and deprogramming the dog in the simplest, most effective way. But this technique will work only

if every time he masturbates, he gets locked in the bathroom and every time you let him out, you do so without
making a fuss over him.

Many people think spaying and castration are unnat-
ural. To some young men, the thought of their pet's castration could symbolize a fear of their own castration. But
castration is often a prudent step to take. If you do not cas-
trate a male cat, he will develop a ghastly odor, a secondary
sexual characteristic, and leave his urine here and there as
his calling card. An unspayed female dog will draw dogs for
miles with her powerful odor. The basis of your choice
should be its appropriateness for your life, not your unexor-
cised fears.

If, as I proposed earlier, we actually create our pets and
their problems, pets can often reveal their owners' sexual
hang-ups with startling clarity.

One woman insisted I spay her dog. Something in her
voice suggested that I should ask more questions before
performing the operation. The woman was terrified of
being raped. She kept imagining all those brutish
German shepherds smacking their lips and taking her little poodle. She told me so. The idea of dogs sniffing her
dog sent shivers through her. I advised her not to have
the dog spayed—thinking that if she did, she would not
be able to play out this fear and be done with it. I understand she went to another veterinarian and had the operation performed.

Once an unmarried twenty-eight-year-old man, visibly
upset, brought in his male dog with a variety of strange and
potentially serious-sounding symptoms. As I examined the

dog, the man nervously told me that the dog had broken free one night and had relations with a neighbor's mutt. The dog had all the symptoms that, I later learned, the man's mother had told him accompanied venereal disease. She had told him about the symptoms many times. The dog did not have venereal disease; he was not, upon close examination, ill at all.

A mother and her ten-year-old daughter came in one day with their black-and-tan beagle cross. They thought the dog was pregnant. The young girl was excited, expectant, hopeful; the woman was terrified.

The dog *looked* pregnant, but I could feel no puppies inside her. x-rays are conclusive when there is some doubt. Here they revealed that this was a false pregnancy, pseudocyesis, a condition in which animals imagine they're pregnant and display all the proper symptoms, including production and secretion of milk. After two months some will actually go through an imaginary birth experience and then try to nurse and protect an old shoe or slipper.

The little girl looked at me, wide-eyed; the mother frowned. "Nope," I said, "she's not pregnant."

The mother let out a long, loud sigh of relief. The daughter said, "But she's been practicing nursing the cat!"

Some months ago, Miss McQuaid, a quiet forty-year-old woman, brought in her chronically constipated cat. She is an extremely proper woman, a registered nurse as crisp-looking as a cracker, diligent, responsible, her bleached-blond hair swept up with every strand in place.

Constipation is common in older cats, and it often requires the removal of the feces with forceps, a horrendous job. I perform the procedure without general anesthesia, and over the years I've found it curious that though cats fuss a bit, they never scratch me while I work. Do they actually like it?

Miss McQuaid said, while I examined Puss, that the medication had stopped working. Then, casually, she happened to mention that the only thing that helped was manipulating the stool out digitally.

So that was it, I thought. The little devil!

A finger up a rectum certainly lets an animal know you're there and it certainly expresses relatedness.

I put on a plastic glove and rammed my index finger—rather than the pinky I usually use for cat rectal exams—up Puss's rectum. It should have hurt her, but instead the cat opened her claws, closed them, looked over her shoulder at me, and said

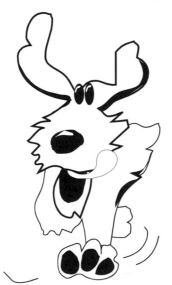

with unmistakably warm and perky eyes, *Oh, you love me, too!*

One need only read half a dozen stories by D. H. Lawrence to know that the desire to dominate is one facet of the Sex Game. For years I've watched men and women come into my office with especially large dogs of the opposite sex whom they control with startling authority. A typical case was the twenty-three-year-old woman who came in recently with an immense, really tough boxer named Alfie. She showed strength and discipline in every gesture she made, every word she spoke, and she controlled

Alfie with the slightest flip of her finger. The dog was per-haps the best groomed, best-behaved animal I've ever seen. The woman had merely to look at the huge dog—who was capable of taking a person apart—and he became her ser-vant. She must have spent hours upon hours training and brushing the dog.

Do this woman and the others like her I've seen want to experience dominance over a brutish male figure? Could such a figure represent their fathers? I have seen many stern, intelligent, sometimes opinionated people who, through sophisticated techniques, have learned how to con-trol such massive animals. They all tend to spend great quantities of time brushing, cleaning, grooming, training, as if to say, "If I do this, he will love me. And if I train him, he will respond to me the way I want him to—the way I wish Daddy had."

CHAPTER 17

The Violent Pet

"HE BITES!" A remarkable number of people have told me that when they bring in their pets. "Be careful. He's a bad dog," they caution me.

When I look at the owners' hands, I can often see that they are right. These dogs have found the ultimate squeaky toy — human hands. They have been playing a bad game.

Of course the problem is more complicated than that. Some owners are perfectly terrified of their own pets; some who have come to me for fifteen or twenty years seem uncanny in their ability to "choose" pets who will bite, scratch, or even maim them or their friends. I knew one man with a hostile, vicious Welsh terrier who bit everything, including his owner's nose. I had to frighten the man into putting the dog to sleep; the terrier was a monster.

Do such people *need* a pet that will tyrannize them? Why, I've asked myself a thousand times, do people want to keep dogs they're afraid of? It can only be that they see themselves, they've re-created themselves, in such a creature. They experience themselves as nice people with feelings of aggression and anger inside them, and they tolerate the dog as they hope the world will tolerate them.

Some owners are perfectly terrified of their own pets; some who have come to me for fifteen or twenty years seem uncanny in their ability to "choose" pets who will bite, scratch, or even maim them or their friends.

Violent dogs are made, not born.

Doberman pinschers are supposed to be like loaded guns. They terrify people. But I haven't seen a nasty Doberman in twenty years; they're big marshmallows. You can train any dog, even a cocker spaniel, to be a watchdog.

I suppose if I were so inclined—which surely I am not—I could even train that cream puff Hildy to be a biter.

Vicious dogs are sometimes created for specific purposes—police work, tracking, or guard work. German shepherds are often chosen for such jobs because they can enforce their anger with bigger leaps, better teeth for the job, and awesome looks; but they are not, by nature, vicious. The kind of angry, hostile, or violent dogs of any breed I have seen in my office have been created by their owners to reflect forces inside themselves that they can't express in a social context.

Whatever the reason they have been programmed to act the way they do, vicious dogs are dangerous. But the programming might only be skin deep. Underneath it is I love you, the basic nature of the dog I needed to connect with.

One guy bought a huge mutt for a specific purpose: to prevent anyone from coming into his apartment and robbing him again. He meant it. He created a monster of a dog, a violent creature whom I was supposed to try to deprogram—and quick! Sometimes I can't and have to say so.

Other "monsters" are all show. The owner brings Brutus in on a leash, and I can hear the dog at the other end of the hospital shouting, *Arrrh, arrrh! Hold me back! Don't let me at him! If I get near that quack, I'll rip his nose off!* And the owner restrains the dog and tells me, "Careful, now. Watch out. Brutus is dangerous." And I suspect the man absolutely loves the image of himself as the owner of this unmitigated terror. With Brutus on the leash, the owner is a real threat. And Brutus learned early in life that if he goes *Arrrh, arrrh!* and snaps his jaws a little, he'll get what he wants. How many people do you know who are just like Brutus?

But when I look at the dog, I suspect he is a fraud, so I walk over, nod, look the dog in the eye, and talk steadily to him. *Hold me back! Arrrh! Arrrh!* shouts the dog.

"All right, chew on this," I tell the animal and put my finger in his mouth.

"*Arrrh. Hold me . . .* the dog starts. *Arr . . . arr . . . aw, my God, it's all over. He knows I'm not for real. He's called my bluff.* And the dog, embarrassed down to his hind paws, can't get out of the off-ice fast enough. For years he's been running the family with that act.

I've had enough cats who act like that, too: all claws, teeth, and ferocious sounds, but no real meanness. The owner of one had been forced to wear gloves. The cat was master of the household. He'd been winning by being ferocious, and though he never actually bit or scratched, he felt obligated to continue the bluff.

Nino doesn't bluff.

Nino is a massive German shepherd, full of dust and sand, who lives in a brickyard. He's totally unruly. He's nearly destroyed people. Recently he bit off a couple of fingers that a kid stuck through the fence on a dare. He means it when he growls.

One day two workers from the yard brought him to me in the back of a dusty dump truck. Nino needed his booster shots (he's never sick). *Arrrh! Grrr-arrrh,* he snarled as they brought him toward the door. *Let me at them. All of them. Anyone. I'm Nino. I'm a killer.*

They had kept him in the truck until his turn, unwilling to risk the lives of anyone in the waiting room. Then a swath opened in the room as Nino lunged forward. There was a spiked collar around his neck, and the two workers, in stained, sleeveless T-shirts, were holding him back with two chains big enough to anchor the *Queen Mary.* The chains were wrapped around gloved hands; muscles bulged in the men's arms. Mrs. Rosenberg picked up her neurasthenic schnauzer and clutched him in her arms; Mrs. McGill's terrier scurried behind a chair. Nino was twisting, turning angrily from side to side. His teeth looked as if they were nine inches long. *I'll chew him up!* he snarled. *Give me ten minutes with this guy and there will be nothing left but his jawbone. Grrr-arrrh !*

The men managed, somehow, to get the dog into the corner of the examining room.

"Nino's a menace, Doc. Don't take no chances. Shoot him with a dart if you got to."

"Hey, dope," I said to the dog. "It's only me. Remember? We're friends. You know you're positively lovable." And Nino wagged his tail, an action that looked more natural on him than the monster mask, came over to me, and started licking my hand.

I knew this dog. What he wanted more than anything was a little love, but he'd been conditioned to believe that the only way to get acknowledgment was usually by being crazy, violent Nino. That's what everyone seemed to expect of him. His job was to protect the brickyard. He got paid, when he acted the part, with recognition. He'd bite anyone's hand—even mine—to get recognition. He knew his place on the sphere and how to stay there.

He got what he really wanted for those few minutes he was in my office—but they were not enough. He was too well programmed. As long as I had Nino's undivided attention, I knew everything between us would be fine. But if the owner was there and said one word, I had to watch out. Nino would immediately think, *Act the other way. The way he wants you to act. That's the boss's voice. I know what I've got to do to please him. This is fun, being sweet Nino—but* mean *is where it's at.*

When I'd hear Nino's owner say abruptly, "Be good, Nino," I'd back off and become genuinely frightened. Someday that dog will kill someone. He turns on and off like a machine and the owner has his finger on the button that makes him go.

> *As long as I had Nino's undivided attention, I knew everything between us would be fine. But if the owner was there and said one word, I had to watch out.*

"I'll handle this dog," I'd have to tell the owner, "only if
you swear you'll be absolutely quiet." I need to get that assurance before I go near Nino and other dogs like him.

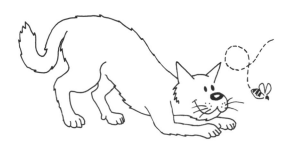

Pets can
indeed be violent.
They have killed,
and they have had
to be killed. One
dog recently turned
on a newborn
infant; another had to be shot down when it attacked a night
watchman. Sometimes their violent game, a bad game, can
lead to no other end. A really bad game cannot be tolerated.
The violent dog may be winning his game but he will surely
wind up dead.

Sadly, somewhere in the history of a violent dog who
plays such bad games, there's always a human being who created such a creature, who made this dog the way he is for
some purpose of his own.

CHAPTER 18

Death

RICHARD, A TWENTY-THREE-YEAR-OLD YOUNG MAN, brought
in a shepherd cross who belonged to his parents. The dog weighed
about seventy-five pounds and had developed two big breast
tumors, large, soft balls that easily weighed fifteen pounds each.
Richard had grown up with the old dog and loved her deeply. I
could see how upset this young man was.

How could his family have allowed these growths to develop to
this size without seeking treatment earlier? I wondered. How
unconscious could they be? I was furious and told Richard so. He
told me his father was in the hospital suffering from a severe
chronic disease. The family had simply been too preoccupied.

"Do anything you have to do," the young man told me. "Expense
is absolutely no issue. We all love the dog." I knew the family didn't
have much money.

I operated on the tumors, which were malignant, and got
exceptionally good results. The dog's breasts healed perfectly, and

six months later there was not the slightest sign or threat of any recurrence. It had been a terrible situation, and the family, who had much else on their minds, were extremely grateful.

Then, approximately one year later, Richard returned with the dog and said, "It's back."

I put the dog on the table and saw at once that one tumor was indeed back—and with a vengeance. It was larger than either of the original growths, a mass the size of a football.

"When did it first appear?" I asked, wondering again how anyone could allow such a tumor to appear without seeking immediate treatment.

"It just got this way a few weeks ago," he said. "My father went back into the hospital two weeks ago and it just grew."

Could this be a coincidence?

From the size of the tumor, I knew I'd have to take an x-ray immediately. There was a distinct possibility that the lungs were affected, and if this proved to be true, there would be no sense in operating because the dog would be sure to die soon.

I told Richard we'd have to take the x-ray, but he didn't understand why. I explained that if the malignancy was in the dog's chest, her lungs, there would be no point in prolonging the dog's pain. He nodded soberly.

I told him to go out and get some coffee. I'd be finished in about an hour, and we could discuss the x-ray results then. He came back while the x-rays were still being developed and before I could say a word asked, "If it's in the chest, it would be best to put her to sleep, wouldn't it?"

Somehow, by the tone of his voice, the nature of his words, I knew at that moment that the x-ray would be positive. Richard *wanted* that dog put to sleep. I suspected, with my knowledge of how much and for how long his father had suffered, that Richard wanted his father put to sleep, too, but I doubted that he could face the thought. Had he, for this reason, re-created the drama in his dog? We were approaching a very difficult moment.

Over the years I have faced death or impending death many times in my office and have thought about it deeply. I was dealing with death again. I knew this now, and I wanted to be as helpful as possible to the young man.

Sometimes there's a question mark about chest x-rays; the evidence is not conclusive, and the negatives have to be examined several times. My attendant brought out the dog's x-rays and a first-grade student would have looked at them and said, "What's that?" There were three prominent masses in the dog's chest. There was absolutely no hope.

I called the young man in, sat him down in my private office, and said, "Look, it's hopeless."

"Well," he said without emotion, "we'd better put her to sleep, I guess." And then, a moment later, he began to cry, grew overwhelmed with anger, and slammed his fist down on my desk. In the midst of the tears, over and over, he asked, "Why, why, why does this have to happen to me?"

How, I wondered, as I had wondered hundreds of times before in similar moments, could I serve this young man best? Death is as real as anything. It is also unavoidable and perhaps not really as awesome as most people find it. Since so much of life is one endless resistance to dying, too many people make dying "bad."

Death is as real as anything. It is also unavoidable and perhaps not really as awesome as most people find it. Since so much of life is one endless resistance to dying, too many people make dying "bad."

I try at such moments to get owners to look at the situation as clearly as possible. I allow them to be appropriately sad; an owner would have to be exceptionally cold *not* to feel sad after sharing a life with an animal for ten or fifteen years. I try to share the sadness with them.

One animal I examined was suffering from an advanced malignancy, a lymphosarcoma, and had no more than three months to live. I told the owners that he was still enjoying life. He wasn't thinking, *Oh, I'm going to die.* I added, "When the time comes, I will help him to die as painlessly as possible." I use euthanasia sparingly, but it has its place in veterinary medicine.

I said to Richard, "If the choice is to end the suffering or prolong the suffering, I have to go with ending it. I watched my own father die from a malignant tumor for sixteen weeks. If I'd had a choice, I'd have ended his suffering earlier."

Richard cleared his eyes and looked at me carefully. I could tell that the drama with the dog was becoming something that would allow him to understand his feelings about his father's illness.

"Sometimes, Richie," I said quietly, "it's all right to want something dead. There's no evidence, is there, that dying is bad?"

He shook his head.

"Remember when your dog was a puppy? Remember how happy and playful she was then? Maybe, just maybe, after death she'll be somewhere doing the same things. The dog has filled you with memories that will always remain with you. She's added to all your lives. And now it's time for an end."

We continued to talk for another ten minutes, quietly, thoughtfully. He asked some questions. I gave him the most sincere answers I could. He mentioned his father and I told him a bit more about the circumstances of my father's illness and death. I felt distinctly that Richard was building, through his dog's terminal illness, some equipment with which he could handle his father's imminent death.

"What should I do for my mother?" he asked suddenly. "Should I get her a new puppy right away, maybe even now?"

I have been asked that question a thousand times. "No," I said. "Don't do that. Let her experience the full measure of sadness. Let her get finished with her sadness over this dog's death. If you don't allow her to experience this, she will be experiencing the new puppy through her unfinished feelings about the death of this dog, and it's quite possible she'll anticipate the new dog's death constantly because she won't yet have gotten through with this one's dying. Let her complete the experience, Richie. Let her strong emotions subside. Then, after some weeks or months, when you think it is appropriate, you can replace her sadness with the pleasure of a new pet."

> *I could tell that the drama with the dog was becoming something that would allow him to understand his feelings about his father's illness.*

I wanted her to experience that combination of grief and emotional relief that comes from a wake or from sitting *shiva*. I wanted her to put a lid on the experience of this dog's death. Otherwise, she might well make a new dog sick so she could re-create the same drama. I wanted nothing to stand in the way of her fully enjoying that bouncy, frisky creature I've seen so many owners bring in for the first time—a new puppy.

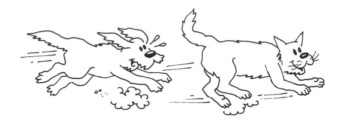

CHAPTER 19

Unity

YOUR PETS CAN—and should—enrich your life. The destructive aspects of the Pet Game often stand in the way of such satisfaction, and knowing the rules and dynamics of the game is the surest first step to greater unity with your pets. If you know the game your pet is playing, if you know your role in initiating or abetting it, the game may still continue—but on your terms. You will not be the victim of the game as much as, consciously, its master of ceremonies. There is a vast difference.

We think that all we add up to are our problems, that we are nothing without them. This is hardly so. Freeing ourselves from them, we have more time and emotional space to be truly creative in our relationships with the world. Remember, *loving something is letting it be what it is and*

> *Remember,* loving something is letting it be what it is and not forcing it to be what it is not. *If you own a pet, you must let him be what a pet is.*

not forcing it to be what it is not. If you own a pet, you must let him be what a pet is. Part of having a pet is seeing a mess on the living room floor once in a while; part of it is an animal's body odor, shedding, scratches on the furniture, a broken object or two—and some games. The process may be uncomfortable at times. But it's also a joy.

Ultimately, what we want is unity. If we can see ourselves in our pets, we can see ourselves better. If we are genuinely one with our pets, we are no longer Herb Tanzer over here and Hildy over there. We learn the pleasures of participating in the life of another creature.

I was remaking my old goat pen one day and had just torn apart the wooden fence. Suddenly I became aware of three tiny baby mice, no longer than the first joint of my thumb. They had no hair on them and could not have been more than a few days old. Obviously, I had torn their nest asunder. My heart sank. What had I done?

I picked the three of them up and looked at them, helpless in my hand. Two were wiggly, pink-nosed little darlings with their eyes still closed tight; the third had been injured and was dying. What would happen to the other two now?

I looked around me. There, five feet from my shoes near a stump, was the mother. The little gray field mouse looked me right in the eye.

I put the three babies down in a row. The mother looked at me steadily, then came right up until she was at my feet. Gingerly she picked up one of her infants and carried it to a nearby stone wall. I stood relaxed in the same spot watching the mouse's every move, trying to let her know my feelings, trying to know hers.

For a moment I *was* that mouse. I knew her fears and instincts, I shared her concern, and I felt her courage.

A moment later she came scampering back, looked up at me again, picked up the second infant, and took it to the same spot in the stone wall. Again, as I stood there unmoving, she returned, looked up at me, looked at the third little mouse, realized it was dead, and returned to the wall.

Mice don't act that way. But this one, somehow, had felt that she was safe with me. I must have conveyed my own feeling of total identification with the mother, of oneness with her. It was a remarkable experience.

Such intimate, warm, knowing, and conscious relationships are possible with pets. But I suspect that a person must be at a certain place in life, spiritually and psychologically, to own a pet and truly experience the satisfaction of doing so. At the time Hildy came into my life, I was able to say, "I am where I am. I like it here. I want a special pet in my space with me."

Hildy is a joyous dog to live with because we do not resist her. We make it all right for her to do anything, which she usually does. Well, *sometimes* she is a joy.

The day after she brought us the pincushion, with its implied threat, my wife had to come to work with me again.

This time Hildy brought out a pair of *scissors*.

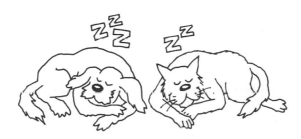

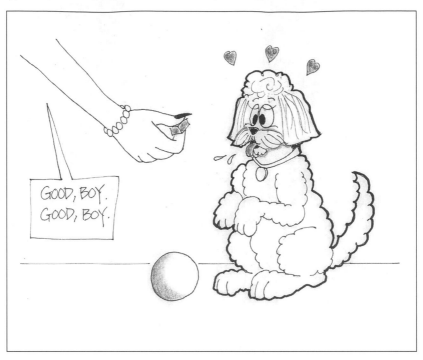

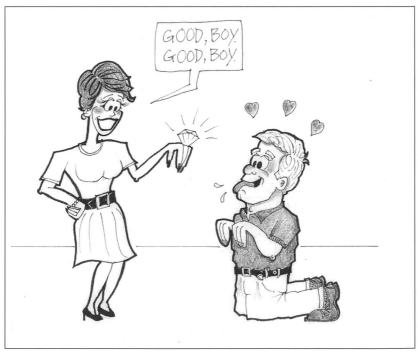

If you want to train your husband,
Buy a book on raising puppies